ARTEM KUDELIA PHD

Psychedelic Therapy

The Healing Power Therapeutic Journeys

First edition

This book was professionally typeset on Reedsy.
Find out more at reedsy.com

Contents

Preface

This vector of psychotherapy encompasses specific treatment methods for neurotic and psychotic patients, utilizing a combination of various verbal and somatic therapeutic modalities along with substances that alter the state of consciousness. Currently, psychedelic methods are very rarely employed in practice. The vast majority of substances used in these treatments are classified as narcotics and fall under Category A, which means they are considered substances that cannot be used in medical practice. However, some countries and certain symptoms make exceptions, allowing for the application of psychedelics. For example, in Austria, the legal use of LSD-25 for pain management in stage-four cancer patients is possible.

Nevertheless, this kind of attitude towards psychedelic treatment methods was not always present in the medical field. Therefore, in order to fully explore this topic, it is necessary to trace the history of the emergence and development of this psychotherapeutic vector.

Acknowledgments

I would like to express my gratitude to my psychology and psychotherapy teachers, who have opened the path and laid a solid foundation of knowledge. Furthermore, I extend my immense appreciation to patients, colleagues, friends, and all individuals who directly or indirectly contributed to the writing of this book.

BONUS: Get Your Free Resources Now

I'm excited to share a **free eBook** and **exclusive access** to **psychological resources** with you. To get started, scan the QR code or visit psychemaster.com/psychedelic-therapy

What You'll Get:

- **Free eBook**: Explore advanced psychotherapeutic techniques and approaches that complement the insights.
- **Interactive Learning**: Engage with exercises and quizzes to solidify your understanding of complex theories.
- **Latest Research**: Stay updated with the most recent findings in the field of psychotherapy and integrative therapy approaches.
- **Continuous Support**: Get consistent tips, strategies, and motivation to assist you in staying focused and excelling in your studies and practice.

Maximize your understanding of psychotherapy!

LSD Therapy

It is best to start with the year 1938, when Austrian chemist Albert Hofmann, working at the Sandoz chemical-pharmaceutical laboratory in Basel, Switzerland, synthesized a significant number of different alkaloids from the parasitic fungus called ergot, which grows on wheat spikes. This plant was often used in folk medicine, and its decoction was administered to women in labor to stimulate contractions before childbirth. During his work, Hofmann tested the obtained alkaloids on laboratory mice, but the results only provided a conditional understanding of the substance's influence on them. In 1938, Hofmann did not find anything particularly interesting among the laboratory material obtained and set it aside in the archives. Five years later, he felt the desire to return to the research on ergot and conduct several tests. He selected one alkaloid that he considered most suitable for testing and began performing specific analyses.

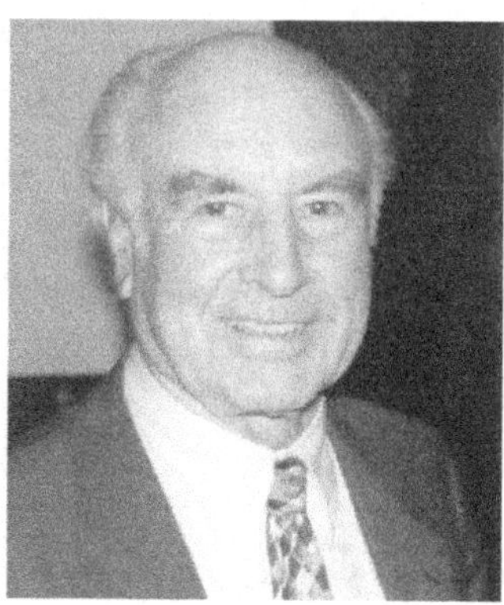

Albert Hofmann

After some time, he began to feel unwell and decided to return home. He left the laboratory, got on his bicycle, and started his journey. As he rode, his condition became increasingly strange and unusual. Numerous sensory distortions started to appear in his consciousness. Hofmann couldn't comprehend what was happening to him but began to suspect that he might have accidentally ingested the alkaloid he had been working with. He remembered that he may have rubbed his eye with his hand while wearing rubber gloves during his work with the extracted alkaloid. There was a high probability that a particle of the substance remained on the glove and later came into contact with his eye's mucous membrane. Hofmann eventually made it home. The sensory distortions he experienced were accompanied by various delusional states. In his book "LSD: My Difficult Child," Hofmann writes that he started having delusional ideas, such as that his neighbor was a witch who wanted to enchant him. He also describes his state in detail: "Upon arriving home, I lay down and entered into a not unpleasant, intoxicated-like condition characterized by an extremely stimulated imagination. With my eyes closed, fantastic images of extraordinary plasticity and vividness surged toward me, accompanied by an intense kaleidoscopic play of colors. This condition gradually passed after two hours while I remained stunned."

After some time, the symptoms almost disappeared. The next day, he returned to his laboratory to test the substance on himself again, in order to fully convince himself that yesterday's state was indeed caused by it. He chose the minimal dosage he believed to be suitable—250 micrograms (later it was discovered that this dosage was more average than minimal; LSD-25 can have an effect on a person even at a dosage of 25 micrograms)—and ingested it. As he had anticipated, his state from the previous day recurred.

Hofmann identified the substance he obtained as LSD-25 (diethylamide tartrate of d-lysergic acid). This substance is semi-synthetic and does not exist in its pure form in nature. Hofmann, Stoll, and Troxler describe the formula of LSD as follows:

After Hofmann conducted further experiments on himself with the substance he found, he decided to share his discovery with psychiatrists who, in his opinion, could derive some benefit from patient treatment.

Hofmann contacted the son of his supervisor, Walter Stoll, who was a psychiatrist at a psychiatric clinic in Zurich, and handed over his findings. Stoll concluded that LSD-25 could be promising for further research and conducted the first study involving both healthy volunteers and mentally ill patients. Stoll published the findings of his research in 1947, which caused a sensation in the scientific community and sparked a wave of new LSD-25 studies in various countries around the world.

The majority of LSD-25 research was related to the "model psychosis approach." The fact that even microscopic doses of 25 mcg of LSD-25 could already slightly alter a person's state prompted the emergence of the biochemical theory of schizophrenia and other psychotic disorders of personality, as well as behavioral and thought disorders. Various hypotheses were formed, suggesting that the onset of the schizophrenic process could be attributed to different endogenously synthesized substances or even specific metabolic cycles. One of the most notable hypotheses was the serotonin hypothesis, proposed by Woolley and Shaw. The key aspect of their hypothesis was the assumption that the profound influence of LSD-25 on human consciousness occurred due to its interference with the functioning of serotonin receptors in the human brain.

Another area in which LSD-25 found application was self-administration experiments by psychiatrists, psychotherapists, psychologists, and students in these fields. At that time, it was believed that LSD-25 could provide a kind of excursion into the world of a schizophrenic, which could become much more understandable after experiencing it firsthand.

One of the first clinical experimenters with LSD-25 on himself was the Czech physician and psychiatrist Stanislav Grof, who would later have a significant impact on the development of this method of psychotherapy and its dissemination worldwide. Grof writes that he underwent his first LSD-25 session in a clinical setting in 1956. He also comments that he was part of an interdisciplinary team that investigated various consciousness-altering substances in a clinical context. This team was led by Dr. Milos Voitechovsky, who introduced him to the fundamental ideas and methods of working with consciousness-altering substances that existed in psychiatry at that time.

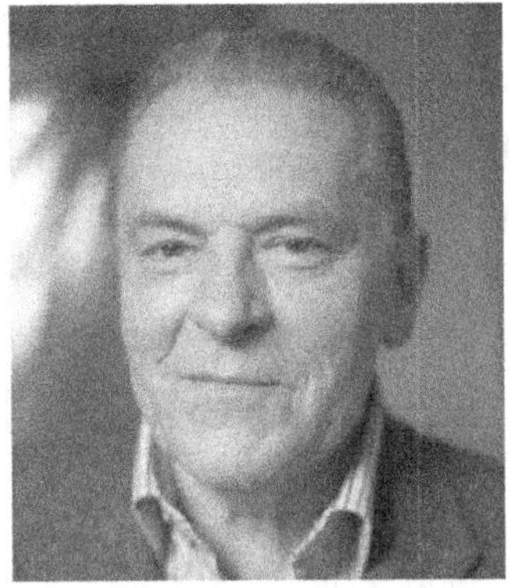

Stanislav Grof

Various attempts were made to classify the category of substances to which LSD-25 belonged. The following names were proposed:

- **Hallucinogens:** substances that *induce hallucinations.*
- **Psychomimetics:** substances that *simulate psychosis.*
- **Psychodisleptics:** substances that *disrupt the soul.*
- **Psychedelics:** substances that *open the soul.* The term was coined by Humphry Osmond. This particular term gained the most popularity and, according to many experts, most fully reflects the essence of the substance's impact on human consciousness.

In 1949, just two years after Stoll's publication on the initial clinical trials of LSD-25, Crowley suggested using the compound as a full-fledged psychotherapeutic agent. In the following years, numerous independent researchers, apart from Crowley, began employing LSD-25 as an adjunct to their psychotherapeutic work. As a result, notions were formed regarding how this compound should be administered, in what quantities, and under what conditions.

After the discovery of LSD-25, the overwhelming majority of research focused on exploring the "model psychosis" hypothesis and its influence on the minds of both healthy individuals and patients with various mental disorders. It aimed to observe how patients with different psychiatric conditions reacted to the compound. Stanislav Grof writes that the pioneers and trailblazers of this research were Frederick in West Germany, Sandison, Spencer, and Whitelaw in England, and Bush, Johnson, and Abramson in the United States.

During the course of working with the compound, many researchers discovered that its use yielded highly successful and inspiring results with patients suffering from the following symptoms:

- Narcotic addiction
- Alcoholism
- Sexual deviations
- Depressive personality disorders
- Sociopathy and criminal psychopathy
- Various personality disorders

In the early 1960s, it was also found that LSD-25 could have an impact on cancer patients. For patients with this symptom, 1-2 sessions of LSD-25 could significantly alleviate their emotional suffering and provide long-lasting relief from physical pain.

Even cancer patients who had no religious affiliations and were atheists could discover a new, profound understanding of death and what might await beyond. Thus, in this case, we can observe how engagement with transpersonal experiences through the use of LSD-25 was capable of transforming the personality of the patient. In some of his books, particularly "The Ultimate Journey," Grof provides several examples of his work with terminally ill cancer patients and the full spectrum of changes they experienced throughout this practice.

The development of LSD-25 therapy was centered in Europe and North America. European psychotherapists established the European Medical Society for Psycholytic Therapy. This society began formulating general guidelines for conducting LSD sessions and developing training standards to prepare psychotherapists to work with LSD. In North America, specifically in Canada, the Association for Psychedelic Therapy was established, with its theoretical framework and application methodology potentially differing significantly from those of their European colleagues.

Stanislav Grof writes that numerous international conferences were held to discuss the peculiarities and specificities of applying LSD-25 in clinical settings. He also provides a list of cities and dates where these conferences took place:

- Princeton in 1959
- Göttingen in 1960
- London in 1961
- Amityville in 1965
- Amsterdam in 1967
- Bad Nauheim in 1968

The 1968 ban on the use of LSD-25 put an end to any further research in this direction and almost any form of clinical application.

Some researchers have suggested that the effect of LSD-25 on emotional and physiological processes in the human body can be compared to the effects of electroconvulsive therapy, insulin shock, or electroshock therapy.

A phenomenon of LSD-25's impact on depressed patients was discovered, wherein they could experience a significant number of euphoric states during the course of their interactions with the compound. Studying this phenomenon, Kondrou proposed the deliberate use of LSD-25 for the treatment of depressed patients, initially employing an approach reminiscent of the old methods of opium treatment. In other words, he administered small doses of LSD-25 to his patients, gradually increasing the dosage each day in anticipation of a psychotherapeutic effect. However, clinical trials with this approach proved unsuccessful. LSD-25 did not exert a direct pharmacological influence on depression.

Subsequently, it was found that the influence of LSD-25 could only manifest itself through proper psychotherapeutic work by the therapist and the patient. It was the targeted work of the psychotherapist that laid the foundation for qualitative changes in the patient's personality.

The pharmacological vector of using LSD-25 was abandoned, and the therapists who explored this topic focused on determining the specific psychotherapeutic work that needed to be carried out during the administration of LSD-25 to facilitate substantial changes in the patient's condition.

Researchers have found that LSD-25 often induces strong age regression in patients, leading them to experience cathartic feelings and release emotions that were previously suppressed. Sometimes, patients would have states interpreted as memories of past incarnations, and such reports were quite common when working with high doses of LSD-25.

The theoretical foundations for describing the findings made by therapists studying their patients' states were largely borrowed from the concepts of Freud and his disciples. These theories postulate that emotional suppression contributes to the development of muscular tension, which conceals unexpressed affective energy. This energy, when not manifested at the appropriate time and place, constantly seeks various ways of release, often manifesting through various psychological, physical, or social symptoms. Once the emotional energy behind the muscular tension is realized, the symptoms arising from the tension should disappear or significantly diminish.

Stanislav Grof describes in his book "LSD Psychotherapy" that at the time of its writing (1979), most therapists agreed that the outcome of a psychotherapeutic session using LSD-25 depended to a significant extent on several non-pharmacological factors, such as the therapist's personality, the setting, musical accompaniment, the conversation between the therapist and the patient, and so on. The compound itself allows for the amplification and manifestation of the processes that already occur in the patient's conscious and unconscious mind.

Grof also writes that LSD-25 qualitatively differs from other drugs in its ability to enhance and expedite the psychotherapeutic process. It is similar in efficacy to several other substances, such as psilocybin, psilocin, mescaline, ibogaine, MDMA, DPT, and some others, which have occasionally been used in clinical practice.

In the context of LSD-25 application in the clinical field, a large variety of therapeutic styles emerged, each differing in their approaches regarding dosage administration, frequency, setting, and manipulations performed on the patient to optimize the quality of work. Here is a list of these styles and their respective creators:

- **Psycholysis** — Ronald A. Sandison;
- **Psychedelic Therapy** — Humphry Osmond;
- **Symbolysis** — Jan van Rhijn;
- **Gebesynthesis** — Harold Abramson;
- **Lyserganalysis** — Roberto Givernetti and Federico Gregoretti;
- **Oneiroanalysis** — Jean Delay;
- **LSD Analysis (Anaclitic Therapy)** — Joyce Martin and Pauline McCririck;
- **Transintegrative Therapy** — Duncan MacLean;
- **Hypnodelic Therapy** — Sidney Cohen and Arnold Ludwig;
- **Psychosynthesis** — Salvador Roquet.

Unfortunately, the majority of materials on the works of these authors are not freely accessible and are challenging to find. Through descriptions of the theoretical aspects and practices of some of them, we can gain an understanding of how these variations of LSD implementation took place in a clinical context.

There were forms of LSD-25 administration where the patient received microdoses ranging from 25 to 50 mcg. During the session, the patient maintained verbal contact with the psychotherapist and freely associated. In this case, the compound was used as an amplifier of the regular psychodynamic process. The primary focus of exploration was the patient's personal, more or less conscious experience. Such dosages often did not lead to experiences of a perinatal or transpersonal nature.

According to Grof, this approach to working with LSD-25 can be combined not only with analytical therapy but also with Jungian analysis, bioenergetic analysis by Alexander Lowen, various neo-Reichian practices, gestalt therapy by Frederick Perls, and others.

Therapists also experimented with applying such low doses of LSD-25 in group psychotherapy. In these groups, all participants, except the therapist, would be under the influence of a small dose of LSD-25. The motivation behind creating such groups was the assumption that accelerating individual personal dynamics with LSD-25 could also accelerate group dynamics. However, as Grof describes, the therapeutic outcomes in such groups were not very favorable. Participants could function adequately in the group only when given microdoses of the substance. Once therapists attempted to increase the dosage, patients would disconnect from the group dynamics and retreat into their own experiences, causing the group to become disorganized.

After some time, this form of LSD-25-assisted psychotherapy was abandoned due to its insufficient effectiveness.

Psycholytic Therapy

Psycholytic therapy, developed by Ronald A. Sandison, involved the use of LSD-25 in doses ranging from 75 to 300 mcg during patient sessions. The term "lytic" in the method's name derives from the Greek word "lysis," meaning "dissolution." The author believed that the goal of therapy was to alleviate tension and resolve conflicts present in the patient's psyche.

LSD-25 sessions were typically conducted once every one to two weeks. The number of sessions varied significantly based on the quality and intensity of symptoms, averaging between 15 and 100 sessions. Psychotherapists practicing psycholytic therapy often shared Freud's views on conscious and unconscious processes, classifying any experience that could be characterized as transpersonal as an attempt to escape the exploration of significant analytical material or as a manifestation of schizophrenic tendencies.

Grof comments that some therapists attempted to analyze the transpersonal experiences of patients and work with them, contrary to psychoanalytic notions.

Grof lists various representatives of this approach to LSD-25 application. In addition to Sandison, they included Spencer, Whitlow, Bakman, Ling, and Blair from England; Andersen-Heyn and Van Rijn from the Netherlands; Johnson from Norway; Hasner, Tauterman, Ditrich, and Sobotkiewiczova from Czechoslovakia.

Many specialists claimed that the main drawback of psycholytic therapy was its excessive duration. Although one well-known practitioner of psycholytic therapy in Europe, H. Leuner, believed that this form of therapy could reduce the duration of the typical psychoanalytic process by at least threefold. It is worth mentioning that Hanscarl Leuner is now famous in the field of psychotherapy for his method of symbol drama, which, naturally, is largely based on his theoretical and practical experiences during the practice of psycholytic therapy. Unfortunately, this fact is not mentioned in any books on symbol drama.

If we compare the effectiveness of psycholytic and psychedelic therapy, Grof writes that no comparative studies have been conducted on this matter. Therefore, on this topic, we can only put forward hypotheses.

Psychedelic Therapy

In contrast to their European counterparts, psychotherapists from North America developed a different approach to the theoretical and practical application of LSD-25 in clinical settings. This approach became known as psychedelic therapy and subsequently became synonymous with working with consciousness-altering substances in clinical conditions. This method was developed based on psychotherapists' observations of patients' experiences, which had a distinct mystical, spiritual, and religious dimension. The creators of this method, Hoffer and Osmond, developed a treatment program for alcoholics using LSD-25 in Saskatchewan, Canada, in the early 1950s. The method drew inspiration from the hypotheses of Ditman and Weitlisi from the United States, suggesting that the effects of LSD on human consciousness and the body bear some resemblance to the state experienced during delirium tremens.

Hoffer and Osmond observed alcoholics who stopped drinking after experiencing delirium tremens. Their initial intention was to simulate a delirium tremens-like experience in the consciousness of alcoholics using high doses of LSD to achieve a therapeutic effect. The results of their tests were quite promising, but it seems that the key transformative element of the intervention was not the simulated delirium tremens experience, but the profound transpersonal experiences that patients encountered during psychedelic sessions. This experiment laid the foundation for the theory and practice of psychedelic psychotherapy, which would later be actively developed and applied to patients suffering from various mental and behavioral disorders.

As the method itself evolved, its key postulates and goals were formulated. The main goal became the dissolution of the ego during peak transpersonal experiences, in which the boundary between the individual and the perceived world fades away. There is a sense of connection and unity with the world and all living beings.

Grof comments that these experiences can be accompanied by visions of the brightest white or golden light, various rainbow colors, intricate patterns, and more. Experiences with various archetypal figures related to specific mythological and religious traditions may arise. Grof also recounts that during his psychotherapeutic practice, he repeatedly observed phenomena where patients, despite not being religious at all, could, under the influence of high doses of LSD-25, have intense mythical and religious experiences.

The dosage of LSD-25 used in psychedelic therapy is significantly higher, ranging from 300 to 1500 mcg. Another notable distinction in psychedelic therapy is the increased attention given to selecting the environment in which the psychedelic session takes place. Preferred settings include spaces that encompass the following elements:

- Beautiful furniture
- Flowers
- Paintings

- Captivating photographs
- Sculptures
- Various natural elements
- Fresh and dried fruits and vegetables
- Various natural incenses

The most optimal locations for conducting sessions are buildings situated near:

- Ocean
- Mountain ranges
- Forests
- Lakes
- Other places that exude the aesthetics of nature

Sound design holds great importance. The space should have a powerful stereo system, and prearranged playlists with carefully selected music should be prepared in advance.

During psychedelic sessions, the following types of music are most commonly used:

- Classical music
- Ethnic music
- New Age music
- Ambient music
- Trance music

Preference is given to musical tracks that either have no lyrics or contain foreign language lyrics for patients undergoing psychotherapy. Verbal communication is entirely halted during the psychedelic work. If the need for communication arises, nonverbal forms of interaction are encouraged.

Grof reports that psychedelic therapy has never been popular in Europe and has been embraced by only a few European colleagues. He also lists notable practitioners of psychedelic therapy in Canada, including Hoffer, Osmond, Hubbard, Smith, Chwelos, Blewett, MacLean, and MacDonald. In the United States, practitioners such as Sherwood, Harman, Stolaroff, Fadiman, Mogar, Allen, Leary, Alpert, Metzner, Ditman, Hayman, and Whitless are mentioned.

Psychedelic therapy has shown its greatest effectiveness in working with:

- Alcoholics
- Drug addicts
- Patients suffering from depression
- Cancer patients

To achieve the full effect, the treatment of symptoms related to psychoneuroses and psychosomatic disorders during a psychedelic session should be accompanied by comprehensive verbal processing.

A significant challenge of psychedelic therapy is the absence of a guarantee that individuals who undergo this form of therapy will have a profound transformative experience. Grof mentions that the effectiveness rate fluctuates between 25% and 78%. He further reports that the highest percentage of transformative experiences was observed in drug addicts, followed by mental health professionals, alcoholics, and cancer patients, while neurotic patients had the lowest level of transformative experiences.

LSD Analysis (Anaclitic Therapy)

This particular application of LSD in patient treatment was developed by two female psychoanalysts from London, Joyce Martin and Pauline McCririck. The term "anaclitic" (anaklinein) translates from Greek as "to lean on something." In the context of psychotherapy, the term refers to the early childhood strivings oriented toward the maternal figure.

The authors of the method primarily used a combination of ideas from LSD therapy sessions at the psycholytic school and supplemented them with their own interesting findings. In contrast to many other psychoanalytically oriented psychotherapists who believe that manifestations of physical contact with the patient can worsen the quality of psychotherapy, Martin and McCririck used excessively close contact with the patient to help satisfy various unmet needs that may have been formed during the early stages of infancy and personal development.

The authors of the method created a new template for the interaction between the psychotherapist and the patient, in which they would be in close proximity throughout most of the LSD session, leaning against each other and separated only by a blanket. The psychotherapist and the patient could embrace each other. Through such "contact," patients often experienced strong age regression, even to an infantile state. When the therapist noticed that the patient had already regressed, they would take a prepared bottle of milk and feed the patient from it, simulating the process of breastfeeding.

The dosage of LSD-25 in anaclitic sessions was relatively small, typically ranging from 100 to 200 mcg. This dose was often sufficient to induce the desired age regression, bringing the individual closer to an infantile state, but not enough to fully reveal the contents of the archetypal part of the person's unconscious. However, it should be noted that the depth of the experience can significantly vary from patient to patient.

Patients who underwent this therapy described their subsequent impressions. For example, they experienced a sense of symbiotic merging with the maternal image. They felt like infants during the lactation process, receiving nourishment from the mother's milk. They experienced identification with the oceanic feeling of unity with the womb. Occasionally, they could engage in experiences with archetypal overtones, where the patient observed representations of mother nature and the image of the Virgin Mary in various cultures.

Martin and McCririck commented that they were able to achieve good results in a relatively short period of time while working with patients with severe neuroses and borderline mental disorders. The authors presented their method at various scientific conferences and even produced a documentary film about it. Colleagues reacted to Martin and McCririck's practice in very different ways, with some expressing admiration and others expressing disapproval. However, the reactions were often emotionally intense.

This form of LSD therapy did not have widespread development and appears to have been practiced solely by its creators. Stanislav Grof mentions his experience undergoing anaclitic therapy with Martin and McCririck and speaks of it in the highest regard, considering it a unique experience.

It is worth commenting on this technique and stating that, in my opinion, this approach can yield excellent results in cases of deep rapport between the therapist and the patient and compatibility of their personalities. Unfortunately, this is not accessible to every patient. It is also important to consider the numerous potential pitfalls that may arise during this type of work. This is particularly relevant when it comes to the potential for the therapeutic process to become sexualized if the therapist and patient are of different genders.

Hypnodelic Therapy

This form of LSD-25 therapy in clinical settings was developed by Levin and Ludwig, combining the administration of LSD-25 with the use of hypnotic suggestion. The name was coined by combining the words "hypnosis" and "psychedelic." During the initial session, the patient's personal history, including significant symptom manifestations, is typically collected and discussed. The therapist also attempted to hypnotize the patient to assess their hypnotizability and the specific behaviors exhibited under hypnosis. Hypnosis was often induced in the old European style using the Lafontaine-Braid technique, where the patient's attention was focused on a shiny object held above their head. If the first session went well, with the therapist gathering sufficient information about the patient and the patient demonstrating adequate hypnotizability, they would reconvene after 10 days to initiate full hypnodelic therapy. Levin and Ludwig typically administered 125–200 mcg of LSD-25 for client work.

Initially, the patient was given a dose of LSD-25, and almost immediately, they were induced into a hypnotic trance to align the effects of LSD and the hypnotic trance temporally. Because the effects of hypnosis do not contradict and often coincide with the effects of LSD, the transition was usually experienced by patients as relatively gentle.

Levin and Ludwig primarily used hypnodelic therapy with alcoholics and drug addicts. According to their observations, combining hypnotic and psychedelic techniques yielded more noticeable results compared to using these forms of psychotherapeutic work separately.

It is also important to comment on the studies by Vogel and Hoffer. In their work, they reported being able to suspend the effects of LSD and induce LSD-like states in patients using hypnosis on days when they did not take LSD.

Group LSD Therapy

This form of LSD therapy is based on therapists' attempts to develop a methodology for working with a group of different patients who take moderate to high doses of LSD-25. There is minimal coordinated interaction between the therapist and patients in this style of therapy. Most often, each participant goes through their own experience independently, although they can interact with each other if necessary. The motivation behind this method was largely rooted in saving therapists' time. During the sessions, participants typically lie down and listen to music as part of the psychotherapeutic process. Different therapists may vary the rules of group interaction.

Salvador Roquet's Psychosynthesis

One variation of collaborative group LSD therapy was Salvador Roquet's psychosynthesis, although Roquet used not only LSD-25 but also various other psychedelics, more commonly of plant origin, in his work. Roquet was unique in combining his psychiatric and psychoanalytic expertise with his deep knowledge of healing practices among indigenous people who had used peyote cactus, hallucinogenic mushrooms, and other substances for ritual shamanic purposes for many centuries or even millennia.

Roquet often assembled groups of 10–28 individuals. The patients selected for these groups came from diverse backgrounds. They could have different symptoms, be at different stages of treatment, and be of different genders and ages. Such a mix was created to facilitate a more comprehensive group analysis process. The more diverse the participants in the group, the greater the likelihood that each member would be able to project the contents of their unconscious and engage in constructive interaction with it. Roquet's patients were often outpatients under his care, and they underwent 10–20 sessions of this type of psychotherapy.

It is also important to note that Roquet's psychosynthesis has no relation to the similarly named psychotherapy developed by

Roberto Assagioli in Italy.

Patients Raised in Families With Religious Fanaticism

Therapists have made a number of interesting observations. It turns out that patients who were raised in families with a lot of religious fanaticism and narrow-mindedness exhibited numerous anti-religious tendencies during LSD sessions.

During the therapeutic process itself, the internal processes in patients begin to intensely project onto the therapists and medical staff. In the eyes of the patient, they may be perceived as criminals, murderers, sadists, perverts, or demonic entities. Conversely, there can also be a tendency where the projections involve the patient's "superego" rather than the "id." In such cases, people in the patient's surroundings may become police officers, judges, prison wardens, or executioners. At times, the entire process of psychotherapy may be perceived as a scene of sexual orgies, a brothel, a harem, a concentration camp, a courtroom, or a death row. Unfortunately, Stanislav Grof, when describing such projections by his patients, does not comment on the specific psychodynamic aspects of their personality that could explain the reasons for the formation of these particular sensory and semantic distortions.

Grof explains that, similar to Freud's perception of dreams as the via regia (royal road) to the unconscious, working with LSD can be interpreted in the same way.

Levels of Personal Experience During LSD Sessions

During an LSD session, the depth of experience can vary greatly depending on factors such as dosage, the severity of personality disorders, the activity of defense mechanisms, the session setting, and the psychiatrist's personality. Grof identifies three main levels of experience:

1. **Psychodynamic Level**
2. **Perinatal Level**
3. **Transpersonal Level**

Psychodynamic Level

At the psychodynamic level, a person confronts deep representations of their childhood experiences. Various problematic situations can unfold and be experienced here. Different complexes can be worked through. For example, a patient may work through feelings associated with the Oedipus or Electra complex, such as fear of castration, envy of the penis, and so on. This level of experience is most often actualized at low doses of LSD. If the dose is too high, the patient may bypass such an experience and delve into the realms of perinatal or transpersonal levels.

Perinatal Level

Stanislav Grof identified four basic matrices of condensed experience that a person can undergo during LSD sessions. He refers to these matrices as basic perinatal matrices (BPM) and numbers them from one to four, according to the order of their emergence. Key experiences at this level involve birth, death, pain, agony, and more. Importantly, these experiences are often not metaphorical but directly felt as real processes. Various sensory and semantic representations of these processes can emerge, such as involvement in combat, being in concentration camps, witnessing accidents and decaying bodies, being in cemeteries, participating in mourning ceremonies, and so on. Significant somatizations can occur. The patient may feel suffocated and experience intense trembling, spasms, convulsions, and severe vomiting. Let's describe all four perinatal matrices that arise at this level of experience.

First Basic Perinatal Matrix

The first BPM encompasses the entire period of the infant's presence in the womb, from conception to the onset of labor contractions. This perinatal matrix is experienced as a vision of paradise, oceanic bliss, and cosmic ecstasy and can evoke real sensations of being in the womb. If there were significant stress factors during pregnancy, the picture may be altered. Representations of cosmic engulfment, a sense of poisoning, and minor spasms can arise.

Second Basic Perinatal Matrix

The second BPM begins with the onset of labor contractions and ends with the onset of the fetus's descent through the birth canal. This experience is directly associated with various adverse experiences that can be interpreted as war, torture, accidents, imprisonment, and physical violence of various kinds. The infant may feel surrounded by various monsters who want to harm them. More often than not, this is accompanied by a sense of helplessness and an inability to escape the problematic context. Scenes of being in hell, confinement in a cage, apocalyptic visions, feelings of inadequacy, inferiority, oppression, pressure, a sense of persecution, and the feeling that the torment will never end, along with ominous mystical omens, can occur.

Third Basic Perinatal Matrix

This perinatal matrix begins with the infant's entry into the birth canal and ends with their emergence from it. The experience within this perinatal matrix is interpreted as a fight, battle, assault, rape, sexual orgy, various combinations of aggression and sexuality, being in a nightclub or amusement park, and a literal reenactment of birth in women. Scenes of murder, bloody sacrifices, and the reliving of death and rebirth may occur. Spasms, convulsions, sweating, and chills can manifest.

Fourth Basic Perinatal Matrix

Stanislav Grof comments that this perinatal matrix begins with the infant's exit from the womb and extends for approximately the first five hours of life outside the womb. This perinatal matrix can be experienced and perceived as visions of vast spaces, spectra of beautiful colors, enhanced perception of everything, a desire to help and support others, and a decrease in pressure. Feelings of grandiosity and manic behavior, as well as sensations such as pain in the umbilicus, fear of death and castration, and severe shortness of breath, may occur.

Transpersonal Experiences

Grof believes that a distinguishing feature of this experience is its specific category, in which an individual transcends the boundaries of their ego and undergoes various encounters with other objects and phenomena. In most cases, individuals deal with experiences they have never had under ordinary conditions or that they rarely experience under special circumstances.

Experiences related to this category can be interpreted by patients as deep regression and exploration of the biological and spiritual past. According to Grof, embryonic prenatal memory can be activated, allowing individuals to re-experience their existence in the form of a sperm or an egg during the conception period. A deeper level of regression can involve transgenerational experiences, where individuals may be associated with the experiences of their family members and witness various fragments of their lives. Grof admits that sometimes these narratives could be verified for accuracy. At times, what a child saw accurately reflected the experiences of their ancestors, even if the ancestors themselves never shared such situations with anyone.

Regression can go even deeper, in which case patients may access their ethnic or collective unconscious. Consciousness can also undergo identification with animal and plant archetypes, as well as various natural phenomena. Additionally, there can be intriguing associated reenactments of organs and cells within one's own body. Many patients are capable of voicing memories from past incarnations. Stanislav Grof provides numerous descriptions of such experiences in his books.

Main Stages of LSD Psychotherapy

According to Grof, the absence of strict time constraints is ideal for LSD therapy. The number of sessions with different patients can vary greatly. Stanislav Grof describes three main stages of LSD psychotherapy:

1. **Preparation stage**
2. **Psychedelic sessions**
3. **Integration of the experiences**

Preparation Stage

This stage involves a specific period of working with the therapist without the use of LSD-25. During this stage, symptoms are discussed and explored using various verbal techniques of psychotherapy. Depending on the therapist's professional orientation, the content of the exploration can vary significantly.

The number of sessions in this stage can range from 5 to 20 hours, depending on the depth and intensity of the issue. A crucial factor is the establishment of a deep rapport and trust between the therapist and the patient, as this can influence the course of the entire therapeutic series. When possible, the patient's personal experiences are analyzed, and key psychotraumatic situations that they have encountered in different periods of their lives are identified. Information about the patient's time in the womb and the process of their birth may also be analyzed if the patient has such information.

Hypnoanalysis can be used to explore important unconscious information if necessary. However, if the LSD session is conducted for self-exploration, seeking inspiration, or professional training purposes, this stage can be significantly shortened and include only a few hours of therapeutic conversation.

Psychedelic Sessions

Grof asserts that ideally, psychedelic sessions should take place in a specially designed therapeutic unit or apartment, preferably on the ground floor. The location should be equipped with a small kitchen and easily accessible bathroom facilities. If the session space is part of a larger working center, good sound insulation is necessary. It is highly beneficial to have direct access to nature, such as a forest or ocean. According to Grof, it is best to start the session in the morning. If it starts later, for example, after lunch, the altered states associated with therapeutic work may continue until late in the evening, causing difficulties with sleep.

Some other psychotherapists, like Mexican psychiatrist Rokuet, the creator of psychosynthesis, followed a slightly different regimen for psychedelic work. Following shamanic traditions of working with psychedelic substances, consumption often began late at night. We cannot provide significant data on the differences in effectiveness between one time period and another.

Grof comments that fasting for one to two days before taking the substance can have several advantages, including reducing the likelihood of vomiting during the session, intensifying and enriching the experiences, and decreasing the chances of negative experiences. If the session is conducted without prior fasting, a light dinner the night before and only a liquid breakfast in the morning before the session is recommended. If the session takes place at a different time, it is better not to consume any food three to four hours before it.

Consuming heavy or large amounts of food can affect the depth and content of the session. This especially applies to the consumption of red meat (beef, pork), which, if taken before the session, may increase the likelihood of negative experiences.

The effects of the substance usually begin within 20 to 40 minutes. After that, the patient is advised to lie down with a blindfold on and remain in that state for the next four to five hours. The schedule may vary depending on the therapeutic school's beliefs and the therapist's personality. The patient wears headphones playing specially selected music. Therapist-sitters are present next to the patient throughout the session, usually one or two individuals. If it is two people, it is recommended to have a man and a woman to fully actualize paternal and maternal transferences. The sitter's goal is to assist the patient when necessary and maintain the most favorable framework for the therapeutic process. It is best to refrain from engaging in any conversations during the session, as it can adversely affect the depth of the experience. Excessive talkativeness from the patient during this period may indicate resistance to the therapeutic process. Communication is only maintained in cases of special need.

Integration of Experiences

After the session, it is recommended for the patient to get a good sleep. The patient can sleep as much as they want. Upon waking up, it is possible to listen to the melodies that played during the therapy session again, and it is preferable to engage in a lengthy conversation with the therapist to discuss various details of the experience. Patients may find various forms of creative self-expression beneficial. Drawing pictures, mandalas, clay sculpting, writing poetry, stories, engaging in dance improvisation, and more can be excellent options. Sometimes, it is through creative self-expression of the re-experienced material that significant emotions can be integrated.

Another technique that can be used for integration is the technique of lung hyper-ventilation. After the legal prohibition of using LSD-25 in clinical settings, this hyper-ventilation technique became the primary substitute for psychedelic work. Stanislav Grof, along with his wife and collaborator Christina Grof, named this form of work "holotropic breathwork."

Usually, hyper-ventilation is used after an LSD session if the patient experiences a blockage in responding to certain residual emotions. When the effects of LSD are waning, there may simply not be enough energy to release some emotionally suppressed products that were not addressed in other sections of the psychotherapy session. Typically, the patient is asked to lie down with their eyes closed, and the music is replayed through headphones or speakers. They are then instructed to breathe as quickly and deeply as possible. This type of breathing usually lasts for 30 to 60 minutes. Often, emotional reactions occur during the process of hyper-ventilation.

Group therapy can be a good choice for working through the experiences obtained during a session with the use of LSD-25.

Psychedelic Therapy with Cancer Patients

Stanislav Grof and his wife, Christina, initially assumed that their patients would be emotionally "normal" individuals. However, they later discovered that this was not the case. Grof writes that at times, the emotional issues of the patients were so severe that he began to suspect a close connection between these issues and oncology. During psychedelic sessions, it was found that cancer patients could have a strong psychological defense that significantly hindered the full unfolding of their experiences. Only by establishing a deep rapport between the psychotherapist and the patient can this situation be changed.

The general content of psychedelic sessions with cancer patients is largely similar to working with patients such as neurotic individuals, alcoholics, drug addicts, and so on. However, LSD sessions with cancer patients have their own specific characteristics, as they tend to be more preoccupied with their bodies.

During the initial stages of an LSD session, various patients may experience nausea, vomiting, tremors, heart problems, and breathing difficulties. In addition to these "common" symptoms, cancer patients may exhibit symptoms indicating a direct connection to the disease and reflecting various deviations that can occur in the patient's body. This can include severe nausea and vomiting in patients with stomach cancer, urinary and fecal incontinence in patients with tumors in the pelvic area, or metastases in the spinal cord.

Grof stated that, based on his observations, LSD sessions were perceived as much more exhausting for cancer patients compared to other categories of patients. They often experience a longer period of fatigue after the sessions.

Grof reports that some cancer patients were able to achieve a sense of self-awareness at the level of their body tissues and cells during an LSD session. Other patients attempted self-healing and the release of emotional blocks in the areas where tumors were growing. In this spontaneous approach to clearing emotional blocks, the foundations of Chinese medicine, which claims that diseases arise due to the blockage of Qi energy in specific areas of the human body, were evident.

Some patients attempted to rid themselves of emotional blockages on their own, while others admitted that they wanted to visualize what they believed to be healing colors. They used colors such as golden, blue, and green. Yet others employed various visualization techniques and attempted to influence the progression of the disease through their internal efforts.

Some participants expressed the desire to complete various unfinished tasks, let go of resentments, express gratitude to their loved ones for what they had done for them, and so on. They could also experience connections with deceased relatives during the session.

Perspectives on Psychedelic Psychotherapy

For over 40 years, starting in 1967, the psychedelic form of therapeutic work was prohibited in almost all countries worldwide. After LSD-25, attempts were made to find a legal substitute for it, but as soon as something similar emerged, the substance would eventually find its way to the streets and be used recreationally within the drug culture. Subsequently, it would be legally prohibited for clinical use.

For instance, a similar fate befell MDMA (3,4-methylenedioxy-N-methylamphetamine) in the mid-80s, which some therapists adapted for working with excessive emotional problems. Although this substance, in combination with therapy, could have an astonishingly positive impact on the psyche, it also had some issues. In particular, it created a regular euphoric backdrop, which led MDMA to become one of the most prevalent club drugs and continues to be so to this day.

Unfortunately, it is true that uncontrolled street use of substances like LSD-25, MDMA, psilocybin, and DMT has led to the prohibition of their clinical application. However, recently (as of 2012), the attitude towards psychedelic therapy in the scientific and clinical communities has gradually started to change. Some American and European psychotherapists have occasionally made attempts to reintegrate the use of these substances into clinical practice.

Additionally, the laws in the United States have been gradually becoming more accommodating toward research involving psychedelic substances. For example, in 2012, during a seminar in Moscow, Stanislav Grof revealed that at that time, students at seven universities in the United States were able to participate in legal research with the use of LSD-25.

Ketamine Therapy by Evgeny Krupitsky

In the Soviet Union and later in Russia, a prominent advocate of psychedelic therapy was Evgeny Mikhailovich Krupitsky (born in 1959). He was the chief narcologist of the Leningrad region, a psychiatrist, and a doctor of medical sciences. Krupitsky also served as the head of the laboratory of clinical pharmacology of addictive states at the A.V. Valdman Institute of Pharmacology, which is part of the I.P. Pavlov St. Petersburg State Medical University.

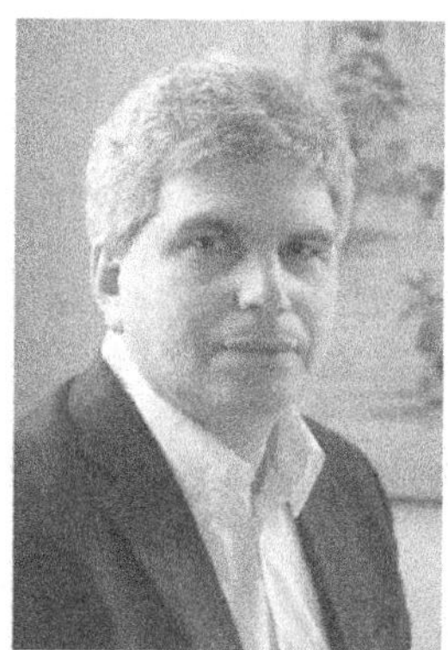

Evgeny Krupitsky

Krupitsky was a member of various international societies, such as the American Society of Addiction Medicine, the International Society of Addiction Medicine, the Research Society on Alcoholism, and more.

The primary focus of Krupitsky's scientific interests was the development and implementation of new therapeutic agents for addictive pathology and the study of the pathogenesis of addiction to psychoactive substances. Krupitsky asserted that significant scientific discoveries were made during the study of psychedelic therapy in the 1950s and 1970s that can be effectively applied in modern clinical practice. He believed that the state of catharsis achieved by patients in the context of psychedelic therapy contributes to positive personality changes and can lead to personal growth and the transformation of one's views on oneself and the surrounding world.

Krupitsky initiated his clinical research on psychedelic work in 1984–1985, using ketamine as the primary medication. Ketamine, commonly used as an anesthetic for anesthesia induction, was employed in exploring the effects of ketamine-assisted psychedelic therapy (KPT) on patients suffering from alcoholism. In the process, he demonstrated that profound psycho-spiritual experiences that could arise in patients during the use of ketamine have the potential to create profound personal transformations. To objectively assess changes in the psycho-spiritual states of his patients, he developed and validated a scale for evaluating changes in the level of spiritual development. This scale was based on the self-assessment scale of spirituality by C. Whitfield, designed to capture changes in the spiritual development of members of Alcoholics Anonymous groups, and the "Life Values Changes Questionnaire" by K. Ring, created to assess changes in values and meanings experienced by patients who underwent clinical death.

During his research, Krupitsky observed three groups of people. The first group consisted of 25 alcoholics after ketamine-assisted psychedelic therapy (KPT), the second group included 21 alcoholic patients who underwent autogenic training, and the third group comprised 35 healthy volunteers who completed a four-month meditation course. Conducting the study, Krupitsky found that alcoholics experienced a significant increase in their level of spiritual development during KPT. Similar changes were observed in the healthy participants who underwent meditation training.

In contrast, patients undergoing autogenic training demonstrated significantly fewer positive changes. Krupitsky discovered that KPT transformed the life goals and beliefs of the patients, effectively influencing their life choices and predisposing them towards a more sober lifestyle. Even in small doses, ketamine enabled patients to access their transpersonal aspects of personality and engage in mystical experiences. Apart from treating alcohol dependence, Krupitsky also examined the impact of ketamine-assisted psychedelic therapy on heroin addicts. However, due to stricter regulations regarding the use of ketamine in the medical field, Krupitsky's research on KPT was discontinued.

Ketamine Psychotherapy (KPT) Method

Ketamine-assisted psychedelic therapy consists of several main stages. Let's list them.

Preparatory Stage

During 1-3 sessions of verbal psychotherapy, patient preparation takes place. The mechanism of undergoing KPT is explained. The patient's expectations, anticipations, and fears are discussed. The psychotherapist informs the patient that they will be able to see, hear, and feel during the psychedelic experience. It is explained that ketamine will actualize repressed and suppressed content in the patient's unconscious. It is also cautioned that the patient may symbolically comprehend the causes of alcohol dependence under the psychedelic substance's influence. This can lead to various insights that can significantly change the patient's life. This stage proceeds as a friendly dialogue between the physician and the patient, creating an atmosphere of trust. The conversation should not adopt an authoritarian or mentor-like tone.

Psychedelic Session

During this stage, the patient is administered intramuscularly with ethimizole (3 ml / 0.10 ounces of a 1.5% solution) to enhance the quality of imprints in long-term memory. Then, a ketamine-containing anesthetic is administered intramuscularly in sub-anesthetic doses (2–3 mg / 0.07 - 0.10 ounces per kilogram / 2.2 pounds of body weight), followed by intravenous administration of bemegride (5–10 ml / 0.17 - 0.34 ounces of a 0.5% solution). Bemegride is used to potentiate emotional experiences and visions. Ethimizole and bemegride also enhance the functional activity of the cerebral hemispheres, significantly improving the quality of the psychedelic session.

Then a musical background is created, which can effectively

enhance emotional experiences. Partial verbal contact may be maintained between the physician and the patient during the session.

The psychotherapist also exerts a specific influence on the patient based on the information obtained during the conversation. The conversation aims to establish a mindset of sobriety and psychological non-acceptance of alcoholism, as well as address specific life tasks that may be relevant to the patient's life. During the patient's profound hallucinatory experiences, the physician may induce the sensation of the smell of alcohol to emotionally and sensorially negate the experience and elicit a negative reaction towards it. The KPT session is always conducted by two physicians—a psychotherapist and an anesthesiologist—in the conditions of an intensive care unit. These conditions are necessary to ensure patient safety, as ketamine administration may lead to complications such as increased blood pressure, respiratory depression, and others. The contraindications for KPT include:

- Endogenous mental disorders
- Epilepsy
- Hypertensive disease of grade II–III
- Ischemic heart disease
- Increased intracranial and intraocular pressure
- Severe renal dysfunction
- Pregnancy

Final Stage of KPT

At this stage, prolonged group therapy is conducted with 4-5 patients who have undergone the psychedelic work. During the interval between the second and third stages, which typically lasts 1-3 days, patients receive an assignment from the psychotherapist to describe in writing, in as much detail and clarity as possible, everything that happened to them during the psychedelic session.

At the same time, they are not supposed to share their experiences with anyone until the beginning of group psychotherapy. This is done to elevate the significance of the acquired experience. During the actual group therapy session, patients share their experiences, comment on various details, and discuss the symbolic content.

The psychotherapist assists patients in interpreting their psychedelic experiences, relating them to their current life situation in general and alcohol dependency in particular. The conversation reinforces the mindset of a sober lifestyle. The psychotherapist strives to help patients adopt a new attitude towards themselves and the surrounding world through the prism of the experience gained during psychotherapy.

Clinical Effectiveness of KPT in Alcohol Dependency Treatment

Krupitsky describes his research involving 111 men suffering from alcohol dependency. The KPT procedure itself was carried out at the completion of a three-month treatment course in a narcology clinic. All study participants were volunteers. The control group consisted of 100 individuals with alcoholism who received conventional treatment methods. The following data on the effectiveness of the KPT method was obtained over time. During a one-year follow-up period, remission was observed in 65.8% of patients who underwent KPT. In the control group, remission was observed in only 24% of patients.

Krupitsky highlights several key elements of the therapeutic potential of the KPT procedure. The first is the associative attachment of the smell of alcohol to the patient during negative experiences that may occur during the therapy session. Krupitsky comments that when alcohol was presented during KPT sessions, patients consistently exhibited grimaces of disgust. The re-experiencing of such aversion at a deep level was fixed in the patients' memory. In this case, we see that Krupitsky employed techniques from behavioral psychotherapy aimed at creating a negative emotional attachment to a stimulus related to the object of dependency.

The second important aspect of KPT is its suggestive potential. According to Krupitsky, during the work with ketamine, patients are highly susceptible to various suggestions that the therapist can create. Krupitsky also notes that the level of suggestibility during KPT is higher than in conventional hypnotherapy. Suggestibility likely increases due to the vivid imagery and intense emotional coloring of psychedelic experiences.

According to Krupitsky, the third aspect of therapy effectiveness is the use of subanesthetic doses of ketamine during the therapy session, which allows for the maintenance of two-way verbal contact between the psychotherapist and the patient. Krupitsky emphasizes that this promotes individualization and a more personalized approach to psychotherapeutic interventions.

Another important aspect is that ketamine enables patients to be more emotionally open and candid during the session, touching upon topics that are difficult to acknowledge in a normal state. This provides an opportunity to influence changes in the patient's values and beliefs, contributing to the formation of attitudes towards taking responsibility for their actions and their lives. Yet another significant factor is the existential orientation of the psychotherapy process, where one of the key elements of influence is the process of meaning-making. This process contributes to creating a foundation for change and transformation in the individual.

Krupitsky also emphasizes the importance of the patient's direct involvement in the psychotherapy process. This involvement primarily applies to the initial stage of therapy and its concluding stage, where patients participate in group psychotherapy.

KPT in the Treatment of Substance Dependence

Krupitsky reports that individual clinical studies indicate the potential applicability of KPT to patients with substance dependence. Similar to working with alcoholics, the method of using small doses of ketamine is presumed to be more effective. This allows for a dialogue with the patient during the therapy session, thereby creating a mindset of abstaining from drug use. Krupitsky warns that KPT should be conducted with caution when dealing with drug addicts to avoid triggering uncontrolled ketamine use. It is necessary to initiate transformative processes in the patient that can change their orientation towards a drug-free life.

Application of KPT for the Treatment of Neurotic Disorders

Krupitsky emphasizes that ketamine psychedelic therapy is not only conducted for patients with alcohol and substance dependence. Pilot studies have demonstrated the effectiveness of KPT in treating various neurotic disorders. The most effective outcomes of psychedelic therapy have been observed in the treatment of depressive personality disorders and PTSD (Post-Traumatic Stress Disorder). KPT has shown slightly lower effectiveness in working with patients with OCD (Obsessive-Compulsive Disorder) and phobic neurosis. The greatest resistance to KPT was observed among patients with hysterical neurosis.

Psilocybin Psychotherapy

Psilocybin and psilocin were synthesized in the 1950s by Albert Hofmann, who had previously discovered LSD. Psilocybin was frequently used in clinical studies as part of psychedelic therapy before it was placed under prohibition along with LSD. These substances naturally occur in various species of mushrooms, and the ritual use of such mushrooms in certain ethnic groups dates back thousands of years.

Among the most renowned scientists and mycologists dedicated to studying psilocybin mushrooms were Robert Gordon Wasson and his wife, Valentina. Another notable researcher of psilocybin mushrooms is mycologist Paul Stamets, who has made significant contributions to reintroducing the medical application of psilocybin through extensive scientific research.

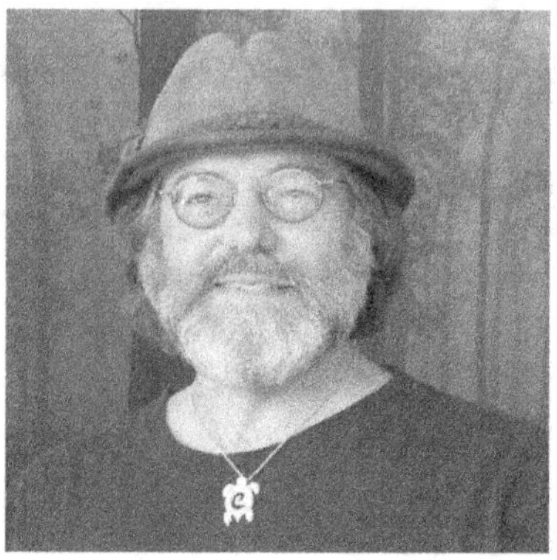

Paul Stamets

Recent studies conducted at Johns Hopkins University have shown that psilocybin, found in mushrooms, can significantly reduce anxiety and depression in cancer patients. Moreover, this effect can persist for up to six months following a single high dose of psilocybin. The researchers emphasize that the findings should not be considered separately from the medical context. It is worth noting that psilocybin is still classified as an illegal narcotic substance in most U.S. states, and any claims about its positive effects can be perceived as drug propaganda. However, it is important to mention that an increasing number of states in the U.S. are starting to legalize the use of psilocybin in clinical research.

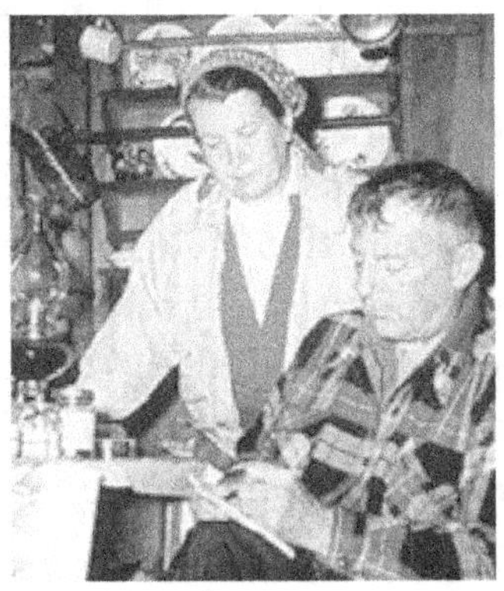

Robert and Valentina Wasson

The next experiment conducted by the Johns Hopkins Institute regarding the use of psilocybin involved 51 participants selected from a pool of 566 volunteers. Prior to the study, each participant underwent a comprehensive psychiatric evaluation. During the experiment, half of the participants received a moderate or high dose of psilocybin, while the other half received a placebo. Over a period of five weeks following the administration of psilocybin or placebo, the researchers observed various states experienced by the participants. Additionally, the participants underwent different forms of testing to assess manifestations of depressive states, attitudes towards quality of life, death, meaning, optimism, and other criteria.

After the completion of the study, the results indicated that the group receiving psilocybin experienced a significant reduction in depressed mood, anxiety, and fear of death, while demonstrating improved indicators of life satisfaction and optimism. In the longer term, approximately 80% of the participants who received psilocybin continued to show clinically significant reductions in depression and anxiety six months later. Furthermore, 83% of the patients reported increased satisfaction with their lives.

One of the researchers involved in this experiment, Roland Griffiths, highlights the astonishingly long-lasting effect of psilocybin, which can persist for several months. Griffiths comments that conventional psychotherapy for cancer patients, aimed at reducing anxiety and depression, often takes weeks or months and sometimes yields no positive results at all. The application of psilocybin to alleviate negative emotional states in cancer patients shows great potential, judging by the experimental data obtained.

MDMA-assisted Psychotherapy

MDMA is a semi-synthetic substance belonging to the amphetamine class and classified as a phenethylamine. It is also known as "ecstasy," "Adam," XTC, and others. MDMA was first synthesized by the German chemist Anton Köllisch in 1914 at the pharmaceutical company MERCK and patented. At that time, the synthesis of MDMA aimed to discover new substances that enhanced blood clotting. However, in the first half of the 20th century, MDMA remained unused in the pharmaceutical industry.

Only a few studies on humans involving MDMA and its derivative, MDA, were conducted in the 1950s and 1960s by order of the U.S. Army under the MK-Ultra program, which aimed to investigate consciousness manipulation using psychoactive substances. After one of the project participants died from an MDA overdose, the research was terminated, and MDMA was once again forgotten.

Its resurgence and widespread use came about thanks to the American chemist and researcher of psychoactive substances, Alexander Shulgin. Shulgin, following a recommendation from one of his students, Mary Clieman, successfully reproduced the complete synthesis of MDMA in his laboratory and began testing its effects first on himself and then on volunteers, gradually increasing the dosage step by step.

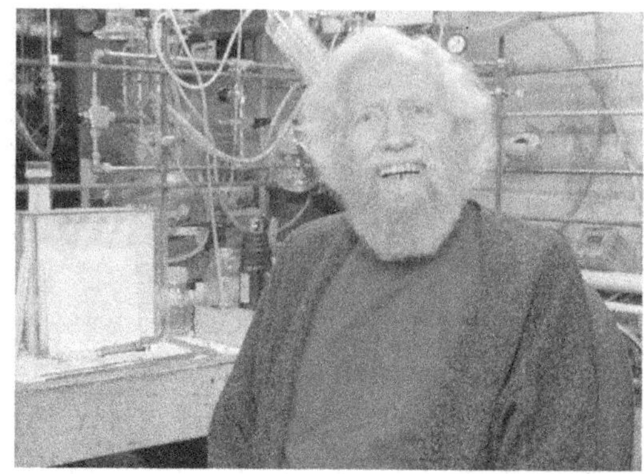

Alexander 'Sasha' Shulgin

Shulgin discovered that MDMA possesses a pronounced euphoric and relaxing effect, gently altering a person's state of consciousness and making empathy and sympathy more pronounced. Individuals were able to vividly recall various forgotten episodes of their lives and express emotions that had been hidden in the depths of their consciousness much more easily.

Shulgin and his wife began attempting the first trials of MDMA therapy with some acquaintances and achieved very positive results. Sometimes, in just one MDMA therapy session, they were able to address symptoms in clients who had been seeing psychotherapists for a long time, often without success.

For instance, Shulgin describes the case of a client who had suffered from severe panic attacks during flights for many years. Psychoanalysis and hypnoanalysis had not helped him.

Key memories that triggered the panic attacks were blocked in his memory. During MDMA therapy, the client was able to regress to his childhood, specifically a moment when he was in school during a lesson. The ceiling collapsed in the classroom, and many children were injured. The client's father was the school principal. After this incident, his father often repeated to him, "We will never speak of this again. We forget about this incident." Thus, the father created a strong hypnotic amnesia in his son regarding the key traumatic experience, which later in adulthood manifested as a fairly serious neurotic symptom resistant to conventional forms of psychotherapy. During the MDMA session, the client was able to deeply engage in the emotional re-experiencing of the traumatic event and express suppressed emotions. According to Shulgin's comments, the client's panic attack symptoms disappeared after the session.

However, Shulgin and his wife were not practicing therapists and did not aim to create separate forms of psychotherapy. Therefore, in the late 1970s, Shulgin decided to introduce MDMA to his friend, psychotherapist Leo Zeff. By that time, Leo Zeff was planning to retire, but after experiencing the effects of MDMA on himself and his patients, he not only returned to full therapeutic practice but also traveled across America, conducting training seminars for other therapists on how to effectively apply MDMA in psychotherapeutic practice.

Leo Zeff gave the name "Adam" to MDMA, believing that this substance could restore a person to a state of innocence that precedes feelings of guilt and shame instilled in individuals during the process of socialization and personal growth. In the early 1980s, many American therapists began actively using MDMA in their therapeutic practices. However, due to the memory of the fate of LSD, which was completely prohibited in the 1960s, the use of MDMA was not extensively publicized in scientific publications and was not widely discussed in public. As a result, no comprehensive scientific studies on the application of MDMA were published, and no research on its specific effects on human consciousness was conducted.

Despite the careful use of MDMA by therapists, the substance extended beyond therapeutic applications. In the mid-1980s, MDMA became one of the most popular club drugs, leading to its eventual prohibition, similar to that of LSD.

In the early 1980s, when MDMA was still not prohibited in America, MDMA therapy showed particular effectiveness in working with patients suffering from post-traumatic stress disorder (PTSD) and depression. It was especially successful in working with Vietnam veterans.

In Los Angeles, at the University of California, full-scale studies on the safety of MDMA use in psychotherapeutic work were conducted from 1993 to 1995. Similar studies were subsequently carried out in Israel, the United States, Canada, and Switzerland. The main subjects of the research were individuals suffering from PTSD, war veterans, victims of sexual violence, and others. Over 130 patients participated in the studies. The research revealed that MDMA has long-term effectiveness in correcting the aforementioned symptoms. However, discussions regarding whether MDMA should be accepted as a full-fledged medication for psychotherapeutic work continue.

Subsequent comprehensive studies on MDMA followed. For example, in 2016, the FDA granted permission for the organization of a large-scale clinical trial of MDMA, which was supposed to involve the participation of 230 patients. The results obtained from this study showed that the use of MDMA in psychotherapy was more effective than placebo by a factor of two. As a result, in 2017, the FDA designated MDMA-assisted therapy as a "breakthrough treatment" for post-traumatic stress disorder (PTSD). Subsequent clinical trials of the method were initiated.

The trials demonstrated greater effectiveness of active doses of MDMA (75–125 mg) in working with PTSD compared to control dosages (30 mg). According to researchers, after the conducted trials, there is a high probability of submitting an application for the inclusion of MDMA in the lists of medical drugs through an expedited and streamlined procedure. The sooner this happens, the better, as PTSD itself is challenging to correct and often leads to suicide, while drugs that effectively heal this condition are not frequently synthesized. A comprehensive decision on the applicability of MDMA-assisted therapy will likely be made in 2021.

Thanks to the active stimulation of dopamine secretion in brain cells, MDMA has the potential to be used in the treatment of Parkinson's disease, specifically hand tremors that occur with this condition. In Parkinson's disease, dopamine levels significantly decrease in certain areas of the brain. Currently, MDMA-assisted therapy for this diagnosis is used unofficially.

In addition to the treatment of Parkinson's disease, oncologists have become interested in MDMA because it has been found that this substance can induce apoptosis in lymphoma cells, and MDMA derivative compounds have demonstrated good potential for chemotherapy in studies.

Ibogaine Psychotherapy

Ibogaine treatment can rightfully be classified as part of the psychedelic approach in psychotherapy, although this treatment method is not widely practiced. Ibogaine itself is an indole alkaloid found in the iboga shrub, which grows in Central and Western Africa, particularly in Gabon. The iboga plant and especially its roots have been used since ancient times and continue to be used in the existing pagan Bwiti cult for ritual purposes. The iboga consumption ritual in Gabon is a spiritually initiatory procedure and is widely practiced in the country. Bwiti shamans have long used iboga and its properties to heal various ailments. Ibogaine possesses strong hallucinogenic properties.

Initially, ibogaine was used in Europe as part of the Lambarène preparation and was used as a stimulant for central nervous system activity and muscle function. It was also used to alleviate fatigue and depression. The use of ibogaine had a place in the realm of sports doping; however, these substances did not gain widespread popularity due to ibogaine's ability to induce deep muscle relaxation after short-term stimulation.

The history of ibogaine's use as a tool in psychotherapy begins in 1962 with a man named Howard Lotsof, who suffered from severe heroin addiction. Lotsof took ibogaine to have a new psychedelic experience, but the 30-hour ibogaine trip yielded very interesting results. Lotsof discovered that after taking ibogaine, he completely lost the urge to use heroin. The desire for it was absent, and withdrawal symptoms were nonexistent, which greatly surprised him. Lotsof began administering ibogaine to various heroin addicts and consistently encountered similar results: a loss of the desire to use heroin and a lack of subsequent withdrawal symptoms. Lotsof attempted to create specific charitable foundations focused on rehabilitating drug addicts using ibogaine but did not find the desired social response and support. Later, Lotsof established the company NDA International, which obtained all the necessary patents for treating drug addiction with ibogaine. The company began rehabilitating drug addicts using ibogaine.

However, by the late 1980s, ibogaine had been placed on the list of banned substances in the United States as Schedule I, causing the company's operations to move to the Netherlands. There, in collaboration with Dutch psychotherapist Jan Bastiaans, Lotsof conducted a successful experiment with thirty volunteer drug addicts. In 1993, the United States Food and Drug Administration (FDA) granted permission for clinical trials of ibogaine, but an unforeseen event occurred shortly after that disrupted the rehabilitation program.

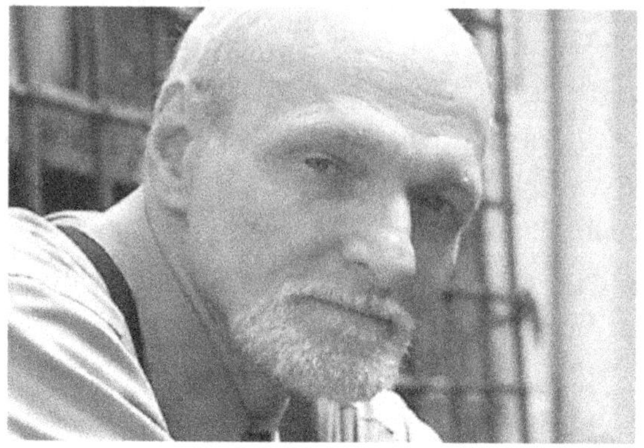

Howard Lotsof

In the Netherlands, during the ibogaine treatment for drug addiction, one of the participants died. Subsequent investigation confirmed that her death was not due to negligence on the part of the leading rehabilitation project. Most likely, the cause of death was the participant's continued secret use of heroin during ibogaine rehabilitation. However, financial disagreements arose between the project organizers, followed by legal proceedings, leading to the closure of the project. Subsequently, ibogaine research ceased, and Lotsof's company went bankrupt.

Despite this, the ideas and practice of rehabilitation with ibogaine found their place in many private clinics, especially in third-world countries, where doctors specializing in addiction medicine began charging significant sums for ibogaine therapy. This therapy emerged in unlicensed clinics in Panama, Costa Rica, St. Kitts, Mexico, and Europe. Prices ranged from $4,000 to $10,000.

Currently, centers that have been working with ibogaine

therapy for a long time have accumulated extensive experience in its application. However, fatal outcomes during therapy did not go smoothly. Over the past 15 years, 12 cases of death due to ibogaine ingestion have been officially registered, and there are serious grounds to suspect that there may be many more unreported cases. Subsequently, statistical data showed that the probability of death from ibogaine intake is 1 in 300.

Since 2007, deaths from this substance have ceased to be recorded. The potential cause of death may be the presence of cardiovascular diseases in patients undergoing therapy. It is worth noting that the ibogaine trip itself lasts for about 30 hours, which puts a significant strain on the heart. Additionally, it should be taken into account that some drug addicts may continue to use opioids during ibogaine treatment, which also ends tragically. The influence of other health-related factors that could not be fully documented and statistically studied should also be considered.

It is important to note that no serious and comprehensive studies on the impact of ibogaine on human body functioning have been conducted. Therefore, there could be numerous factors that contribute to fatal outcomes.

The format of ibogaine therapy bears many similarities to the basic format of psychedelic therapy, where the psychotherapist acts as a sitter in clinical conditions, assisting and providing support to the patient when necessary. Various techniques and practices related to different therapeutic traditions can be employed in the process. It is highly desirable for the therapist to understand the possible experiences and specific emotional states the patient may encounter and to know what actions can be taken in response to those experiences and crises. It should be noted that ibogaine administration can induce strong vomiting and other physiological reactions; thus, the sitter should possess resuscitation skills to provide qualified assistance if needed.

Prior to the clinical use of ibogaine, it is important for the patient to undergo at least minimal verbal psychotherapy in which the psychological issues to be addressed are discussed.

Patients should be informed that the use of ibogaine carries a relatively high risk of fatal outcomes.

Patients with severe mental disorders and cardiovascular diseases are not recommended to undergo ibogaine therapy.

In the process of clinical application, the following information regarding the dosing of ibogaine has been obtained. When using pure ibogaine hydrochloride, it should be administered at a dosage of 10 mg/kg for men and 9 mg/kg for women. In the case of heroin addicts undergoing ibogaine therapy, the dosage should be doubled, as opioids may partially block the effects of ibogaine. It is highly undesirable to consume any narcotics or alcohol at least 24 hours before the ibogaine session, as it may have unpredictable consequences.

At the beginning of the ibogaine intake, the effects of the substance typically start manifesting approximately 30 minutes after administration and gradually develop over a period of two hours. Various bodily, auditory, and visual representations can occur. Tinnitus, coordination difficulties, and heightened perception of sounds and colors may be experienced. Vomiting can occur around three hours after ibogaine intake.

The ibogaine therapy session itself lasts a very long time, sometimes spanning 20 to 30 hours, and in some cases, it may extend over several days. Meaningful communication with the patient during the session can be quite challenging. The patient can drink water, but the consumption of food is likely to be impossible, so it is best to refrain from it.

Two main phases of the ibogaine trip are distinguished: the oneirophrenic and the processive phases. During the oneirophrenic phase, the individual sees a multitude of flowing images and experiences with closed eyes. It can resemble watching vivid and colorful movies. These intense visions often directly relate to the patient's life memories, presented in a direct or symbolic form. This phase typically begins around 1 to 2 hours after the start of the session. The processive phase is a phase of processing and understanding the acquired experience, where cognitive processes and analysis become more active. The onset of this phase occurs approximately 3 to 6 hours after ibogaine intake and can last from 8 to 14 hours.

In many cases, a single ibogaine session is sufficient to induce constructive changes in consciousness and physiology. However, there may be a need to duplicate the ibogaine therapy session. In such cases, it is recommended to maintain a minimum of one month between the two working sessions.

After the ibogaine therapy session, the intake of melatonin and B-group vitamins is recommended.

Finally, it is worth reminding and emphasizing that in West Africa, specifically in Gabon, where the tradition of iboga root consumption originated, ibogaine is used by the shamans of the Bwiti cult as a universal therapeutic and initiatory agent for balancing the mind and body. Iboga "therapy" in Gabon is by no means limited to drug addiction but offers a broader spectrum of correction for mental and physical disorders.

Modern neurological research has shown that the consumption of iboga root stimulates the abundant production of a neurotransmitter in the brain, which has been named "ibogaine." It is believed that the abundant secretion of the ibogaine

neurotransmitter in the brain somehow "overloads" the synthesis of basic neurotransmitters, resulting in a state of balance
in the mind. However, this is just one hypothesis that still
requires verification and validation. For now, it is important
to consider that the effect and therapeutic impact exist, and
further research is needed to determine precisely how ibogaine
affects the human brain and body.

Post-psychedelic Forms of Psychedelic Therapy

After the prohibition of psychedelics in clinical practice, many doctors and scientists turned to developing legal therapeutic methods that, on the one hand, do not involve the use of prohibited chemical substances but, on the other hand, can provide benefits comparable to those of psychedelic therapy. In the context of this book, we will describe three prominent representatives of the post-psychedelic culture who actively worked with individuals using psychedelics before their formal prohibition. These individuals are Stanislav Grof, John Lilly, and Hankskarl Leuner.

Stanislav Grof's Holotropic Breathwork

Stanislav Grof was born in 1931 in Czechoslovakia. He completed his medical degree at Charles University in Prague in 1956 and specialized as a clinical psychiatrist. At the beginning of his career, he primarily focused on the clinical application of psychoanalysis.

In 1959, Grof was awarded the Karel Kuffner Prize for his outstanding contributions to the field of psychiatry.

Grof underwent training in psychoanalysis with Fedor Dosuzkov, his psychoanalytic teacher. However, Grof's psychoanalytic ideas were significantly transformed by his involvement in the clinical use of LSD-25, which was gaining momentum in the late 1950s. While working with patients using this substance, he regularly observed feedback from them that did not fit into traditional psychoanalytic concepts. Faced with this dilemma, he had to choose between considering the feedback from LSD-taking patients as the product of the mind's immersion in a state of profound intoxication, a hallucination devoid of practical value, or regarding the experiences as significant information that significantly expands our understanding of the psyche. Grof chose the latter path and dedicated himself entirely to working with LSD-25 for many years. He defended his dissertation on the subject of LSD's application to obtain his Ph.D. in Philosophy in 1965 at the Czechoslovak Academy of Sciences.

However, following the prohibition of clinical use of LSD-25, he was compelled to seek other means to clinically actualize transpersonal experiences in patients. After some time, Grof, along with his wife Christina, developed the method of Holotropic Breathwork, which, in terms of effectiveness, is similar to the practice of using LSD-25 but with specific differences. Since then, Grof has been teaching the technique and practice of Holotropic Breathwork to this day (2019).

In 1969, Grof became one of the founders of the "Journal of Transpersonal Psychology." That same year, he joined an experiment on the use of psychedelics at the Spring Grove facility, which was being conducted at the Maryland Psychiatric Research Center.

Grof's first marriage ended in 1975. Afterward, he married Christina Hill, who later took his surname. It is with her that Grof has been conducting seminars on transpersonal psychotherapy and holotropic breathwork for many years.

In 1977, Stanislav Grof, along with Michael Murphy and Dick Price, founded the International Transpersonal Association, of which he served as president from 1978 to 1982.

In 1993, Grof received the Honorary Award from the Association of Transpersonal Psychology.

In 1995, he became a professor at the Department of Psychology at the California Institute of Integral Studies.

In 2007, Grof was awarded the title of Honorary Professor by Moscow State University. He also became an Honorary Member of the Russian Psychological Society.

In 2014, his wife and collaborator, Christina Grof, passed away.

In 2016, Stanislav Grof married psychotherapist Brigitte Aschauer, who took his surname.

As of 2019, Grof continues to work, conduct seminars on transpersonal psychology, and contribute to the development of humanity's scientific potential.

Some of Stanislav Grof's most famous books include "Realms of the Human Unconscious," "The Cosmic Game," "The Holotropic Mind," "The Holotropic Breathwork," "Spiritual Emergency," "Beyond the Brain," "Psychology of the Future," "The Stormy Search for the Self," and others.

Stanislav Grof, while observing patients undergoing psychedelic therapy, discovered that their experiences could be categorized into distinct blocks. Part of the experience patients had was directly related to the infantile, or what is commonly referred to as the "Freudian" unconscious. In this case, patients dealt with various childhood memories, unresolved traumas, and associated emotions. Another significant sphere that Grof observed in many of his patients was the realm of prenatal development. He found that through LSD-25 therapy and later through holotropic breathwork, individuals could vividly recall and resurrect in their consciousness various emotional experiences in general and psychotraumatic situations in particular that might have occurred during their time in the maternal womb. The mapping of this experience was so extensive that Grof had to divide it into four basic perinatal matrices (BPM).

We partially explore the topic of BPM in the chapter dedicated to the psychedelic dimension in therapy, where we delve deeply into Stanislav Grof's contributions to LSD therapy. In this section of the book, we touch upon these topics only briefly.

By the first BPM, Grof understood the experiences accumulated by a person during their time in the maternal womb—the entire period of pregnancy before the onset of labor and childbirth. This experience is often remembered as "oceanic bliss" and unity with the "cosmos." Problems can arise if the mother experienced any psychotraumatic events during pregnancy, desired to abort the child, suffered physical trauma, and so on. In such cases, each of these experiences leaves emotional imprints on the child and, to some extent, influences their personality dynamics.

The second BPM occurs when contractions begin, the placenta tears, but the birth canal has not yet dilated. This state almost always leaves strong negative impressions in the individual's consciousness, although the duration of the child's stay in this phase can have significant importance. When recalling such an experience, a person may see images of various beings threatening to attack them, monsters, or the dead who want to torment them, render them helpless, and so on.

The third BPM actualizes the experience of actively passing through the birth canal. A person may recall this experience as passing through a tunnel, the walls of which are adorned with knives and dagger blades. It can be an image of a tunnel, corridor, cave, and so on. In any case, there is a motif of struggle and resistance present. Aggressive and sexual feelings are often actualized during this stage.

Grof identified the fourth BPM as the experience of liberation from the confinement of the womb during the first five hours after birth. Feelings of weightlessness, freedom, and completeness are actualized, and images of carnival processions, grand celebrations, and collective rejoicing may be seen. Sometimes, if the birth was very difficult, the fourth perinatal matrix may take on connotations of sorrow and the process of dying.

The third level of the unconscious that Grof identified, working with the feedback from his patients, was the transpersonal level. The content of this level lies beyond the literal experience of the individual. It encompasses the experience of collective memory of the group to which the person belongs, ancestral memory, and even archetypal content that relates to all of humanity as a whole. Carl Jung referred to this level as the collective unconscious. Here, a person can recall the experiences of their past incarnations and associate them with the experiences of various animals, natural elements, and material objects.

Grof considered these three levels of the human unconscious as systems of condensed experience (SCEs), which, in his opinion, are three key links in human consciousness.

The term "holotropic," which Grof used in relation to the name of therapeutic breathing, can be translated from Ancient Greek as "directed towards wholeness." The technique of holotropic breathing is quite simple and is likely borrowed from yogic breathing techniques (pranayama). In pranayama, breathing techniques similar to holotropic breathing are called kapalabhati and bhastrika. Both types of breathing involve the use of lung hyperventilation techniques.

It is also worth noting that before Grof, Wilhelm Reich, a disciple of Freud and the creator of vegetotherapy, as well as his students, including Alexander Lowen, could have used intensive breathing techniques in their work with patients. However, neither Reich, Lowen, nor their followers made hyperventilation a central technique in their therapeutic methods.

Leonard Orr independently used hyperventilation techniques in the process of psychotherapy and called his method "rebirthing." Currently, it is quite difficult to trace whether Grof borrowed techniques from Orr or vice versa because both holotropic breathing and rebirthing emerged in the mid-1970s. Despite their general similarities, the methods can differ significantly in details.

When working with holotropic breathing, the patient is instructed to lie on the floor on a soft mat and begin breathing intensively through the mouth. There are no strict rules for breathing, but fast and deep breathing is preferred. The faster and deeper the breathing, the more likely it is to induce an altered state of consciousness. From a physiological perspective, during intensive breathing, carbon dioxide is flushed out of the person's blood, and the blood vessels in the brain constrict, leading to the inhibition of the functioning of the cerebral cortex. Additionally, the limbic system of the brain becomes activated, which, in turn, triggers a range of diverse experiences, such as deep euphoria, various illusions and hallucinations, profound inner experiences, and access to bodily sensations that are often inaccessible in the usual state. It is also worth noting that blood pH increases, causing respiratory alkalosis, which is a disturbance in the acid-base balance of the body.

However, despite this, the breathing technique itself does not entail any serious negative consequences for the body, although some critics of holotropic breathing claim otherwise, suggesting that brain cells can die during asphyxia. However, there is no scientific evidence to support this claim. Many practitioners who have undergone tens or even hundreds of hours of holotropic breathing sessions have not experienced any illnesses. Stanislav Grof commented that over more than 30 years of actively conducting holotropic breathing seminars, he has facilitated this form of therapeutic work with over 30,000 people, and the variety of feedback he has received from them can truly be impressive.

The foundation of holotropic breathwork therapy draws heavily from the structure of working with patients in psychedelic psychotherapy. The preferred format of work is group therapy, with the number of participants ranging from 4 to 20, although Grof does not set an upper limit on the number of participants. For instance, when conducting holotropic breathwork seminars in different countries, he has worked with groups consisting of more than 50 participants.

Before the breathing session begins, participants are instructed by the therapist regarding the session itself, what might happen, the specific experiences that may arise, and what to do in case of any negative experiences. It should be noted that depending on the individual neurophysiology of each participant, sensory experiences can vary greatly and may focus on specific sensations.

Some participants may have multiple visual experiences during the breathing process, which may include sensory distortions or sequentially meaningful experiences. Others may place greater emphasis on external and internal sensations, while some may experience increased motor representation of sensations, such as waving their arms and legs, hitting the floor, experiencing vibration, spasms, limb paralysis, and so on.

During holotropic work, some participants may produce various sounds, often reflecting specific emotional states that are not constructively expressed in ordinary states of consciousness. These sounds can include laughter, screams, crying, uproarious laughter, hissing, prolonged vocalization of vowels, and so on. Olfactory and gustatory representations are relatively rare.

Participants are informed that almost any form of sensational expression is a form of emotional release, and it is highly undesirable to restrain these expressions during the breathing process. The only fundamental limitation is the prohibition of directly involving other group members in reacting to one's own emotions.

If the group consists of more than 4–5 individuals, it may be optimal to divide it into sitters and breathers during the breathing session. The sitter acts as an assistant to the therapist and remains next to the breather, providing support if necessary throughout the session, which usually lasts from 45 to 90 minutes. Then, at the end of the breathing session, the sitter and breather switch places.

Sometimes, during the breathing process, there may be a need to work with the patient's body, for example, when excessive motor representation becomes evident. In such cases, when the patient is moving too intensely and cannot control their movements, the therapist may approach the patient and temporarily block their intense movements with their hands or their entire body, allowing the patient to experience resistance and express their emotional response in a more concentrated manner.

In this way, the therapist helps the patient "exhale" more quickly. Once the intensity of the energy begins to diminish, the therapist releases the patient and allows them to continue breathing. Sometimes, the sitter with experience in this form of patient interaction may directly work with the patient's body.

An integral part of the holotropic breathwork session is the use of music. The playlist for the breathing session is often composed of classical and ethnic music, New Age music, a combination of ethnic and light electronic music, ambient soundtracks, and so on. It is undesirable to use tracks with lyrics or songs in the language spoken by the participants themselves. Soundtracks without lyrics or with minimal lyrics are preferable. The fewer semantic associations the patient receives through words in the music, the better. In addition to musical accompaniment, various world incenses are used during the holotropic breathwork session to create a favorable and calming state for the patient. Some therapists may also play various ethnic shamanic instruments, such as the shamanic drum, bongos, jew's harp, didgeridoo, and so on, in addition to the regular musical accompaniment.

As the breathing session approaches its end, the music gradually fades, and participants are asked to lie down for a while, aligning their breathing and avoiding quick movements. When all the patients have returned to a normal state, a group sharing session begins. They share their experiences and discuss the emotions they encountered during the breathing process. Typically, the therapist does not conduct an in-depth analysis of the patients' experiences, although in some cases, specific analytical comments may be appropriate. However, in the holotropic breathwork approach, special emphasis is not placed on analyzing the experiences. If patients manage to access the transpersonal realm of their personality and experience certain archetypes of the human unconscious, the therapist may recount stories from myths and legends that contain the images seen by the patient. Naturally, in such cases, the therapist must be knowledgeable in the fields of mythology and religious studies.

Each holotropic breathwork session can significantly differ from previous ones, offering unique insights, emotional responses, and a specific understanding of oneself, others, and the world. The holotropic breathwork technique itself can be effectively applied as a standalone method of psychotherapy or as a valuable complement to other therapeutic approaches.

77

Hanskarl Leiner's Symboldrama

Hanscarl Leuner (1919–1996) was a German psychotherapist, professor, and medical doctor. He was the creator of:

- Catathymic-imaginative psychotherapy, also known as "symbol drama"
- The International Society for Catathymic Imaginative Experience and Imaginative Methods in Psychotherapy and Psychology
- The European Medical Society for Psycholytic Psychotherapy

Leuner also served as the head of the psychotherapy and psychosomatics department at the psychiatric clinic of the University of Göttingen in Germany. He was born in Bautzen, Germany, into a merchant family. During his studies in Germany, he aspired to become a physician and psychotherapist.

There is an amusing story about Leuner's decision to seek advice regarding his future profession from Fritz Künkel, a renowned psychotherapist at the time in Germany. Künkel ironically told him that in order to become a good psychotherapist, he would first have to complete medical school and then forget everything he had been taught there. Considering Leuner's significant success in his profession, we can assume that he took his "guru's" recommendation to heart.

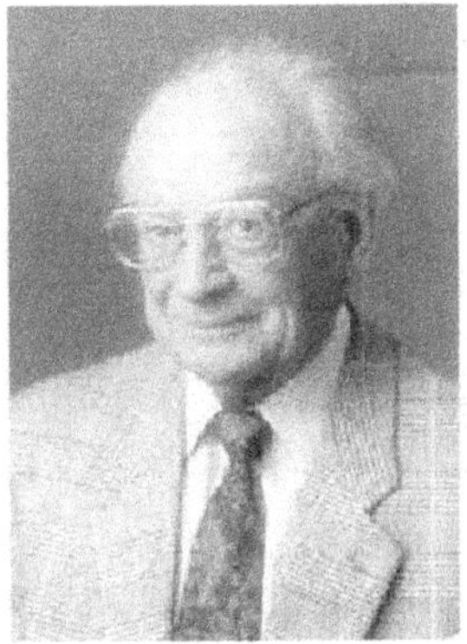

Hanskarl Leiner

In 1937, Leuner graduated from high school. In 1939, he enrolled in the medical faculty of Frankfurt University. That same year, he was called to the front and served as a radio operator in the tank troops until 1941. Due to a shortage of doctors in Germany in 1941, he was sent back from the front to study at the medical institute.

In 1946, after the war, he passed his state exams at the University of Marburg. In 1947, Hanscarl Leuner defended his dissertation. From 1947 to 1948, he underwent training in Jungian psychoanalysis under Gustav Schmalz, who was a disciple of Carl Jung and had himself undergone analysis with him. During that period, the attitude towards Jungian analysis was quite skeptical, as Jung's psychotherapeutic contributions were considered more products of his intuition than forms of scientific experimentation. Nevertheless, Leuner recognized the effectiveness of Carl Jung's therapeutic method and began working on experiments that could validate Jung's theories and make them clinically adaptable.

From 1948 to 1954, Leuner attempted to improve Jung's method. In the process of this "improvement," he developed his own comprehensive psychotherapy method, which was later named "catathymic-imaginative psychotherapy" or "symbol drama." Naturally, this method was rooted in Jungian analysis, but in theory and practice, it differed significantly from it.

In his works, Leuner describes working with the motives of symbol drama, such as "Meadow," "Stream," "Mountain," "House," "Name," "Important Person," "Hitchhiking," "Bog Hole," and "Entrance to the Cave." Additionally, Leuner introduced practices such as working with "fixed images" and "transformation phenomena" into his therapeutic work.

From 1955 to 1957, Leuner developed a practice of working with symbolic beings in the imagination. Its foundation naturally lies in Jungian active imagination practice.

Leuner proposed specific motifs of imagination that could facilitate interaction with these "beings." He would ask his patients to imagine a bog hole or the entrance to a cave. Then, for some time, the patient was instructed to simply contemplate the given motif.

Afterwards, Leuner would give a directive command: "Now, some creature or person will emerge from the hole; observe it." Frequently, the images that appeared in the patients' imaginations greatly frightened them. Leuner referred to this emotional phenomenon as the "horror of the Gorgon."

Despite the intense negative emotions, Leuner encouraged patients to observe the images. Over time, the images themselves became less intimidating and threatening. This therapeutic process took up to 30 minutes of session time.

When the goal was achieved, Leuner would instruct patients to approach the visualized object, touch it, or simply stroke it. According to Leuner, this process allowed for the release of suppressed affective tension in the patient's psyche and the integration of the experience behind it.

In 1959, Leuner began researching the active imagination of symbolism in various landscapes. He attempted to identify specific fixed criteria that differentiated the visualization of landscapes in individuals with different neurotic pathologies from those in a normal state of consciousness. He discusses his work on this topic in the article "Landscape Image as a Metaphor of Dynamic Structures."

In 1959, Leuner worked at the psychiatric clinic of the University of Göttingen, where he led the department of psychotherapy and defended his doctoral dissertation in psychiatry and neurology.

In 1960, during one of the seminars conducted by Leuner, a discussion emerged that subsequently influenced the development of the associative method in symbol drama.

From 1963 to 1973, Leuner continued his psychoanalytic education at the Educational Center for Psychotherapy and Psychoanalysis in Göttingen. During this period, he underwent supervision with Franz Haygler and analyses by Haygler-Evers and Werner Schwidder.

In 1964, Hanscarl Leuner published his article "The Associative Method in Symbol Drama."

During the same year, he founded the European Medical Society for Psycholytic Psychotherapy (EPT). In 1965, he obtained the title of professor. In 1974, he established the Society for

Catathymic Experience of Images and Imaginative Methods in Psychotherapy and Psychology (AGKB). In 1975, he assumed the leadership of the Department of Psychotherapy and Psychosomatics at the Center for Psychological Medicine at the University of Göttingen. In 1978, he created the International Society for Catathymic Experience of Images and Imaginative Methods in Psychotherapy and Psychology (IGKB). He retired in 1985. In 1996, he passed away from pneumonia in Göttingen.

Throughout his prolific career, Hanscarl Leuner conducted numerous lectures and training programs in various cities in the United States and Europe. He was one of the pioneers in the study of LSD-25 and its effects on the psyche and consciousness. He was regarded as one of Germany's leading experts in this field of research. There were various styles of applying LSD-25 in psychotherapy and psychiatry.

The psycholytic method, actively utilized by Leuner, was particularly popular in Europe. Its distinct feature was the use of small dosages of LSD-25 and a large number of therapy sessions. During the psychotherapy process, patients could undergo over 100 sessions involving the administration of LSD-25 over several years.

The psychedelic method gained significant popularity in the United States and Canada, focusing on the use of higher dosages of LSD-25 and a smaller number of psychotherapy sessions, usually no more than ten.

The method of symbol drama spread to many countries worldwide and found its application in various domains of psychotherapeutic practice.

Pathopsychological Profiles and Psychedelic Therapy

When describing the influence of psychedelic substances on patients with different pathopsychological profiles, we specifically mention LSD-25. It is important to consider that the reactions of individuals belonging to specific profiles to other substances may be quite similar. The majority of the statistical data we relied on in writing this work was directly related to LSD-25. That is why we selected this particular substance as a reference point.

Hysteroid Profile

In patients with a hysteroid personality profile, LSD sessions often reveal intense and profound experiences, even with small dosages. Internal sensory representations span a wide range of visual spectra, producing a multitude of diverse images. The behavior of these patients can appear extravagant and exalted. All unconscious processes within the hysteroid personality become more intensified. What would take several dozen psychotherapy sessions to unfold in a hysteroid individual can be condensed into a single session. There is a high likelihood of an erotized transference toward a therapist of the opposite gender, as well as the emergence of numerous fantasies involving the therapist, sitter, or other individuals present during the LSD session. Hysteroid individuals more frequently generate strong and inflated sexual transferences. The patient may perceive the therapist as the embodiment of the "id," such as an Arab drug dealer, a native Aborigine, Casanova, a crime lord, or a great seducer. Transferences related to the "super-ego" may also occur, such as the image of a holy person, the world's best therapist, Jesus, Mohammed, Buddha, a hero saving the world, and so on. Hysteroid personalities, more often than other patients, recall past incarnations, remembering that the therapist had a connection to them, that they have met many times, and so forth. Such patients enjoy discussing these topics, elaborating on the details of their experiences, and withholding nothing. They tend to exaggerate the positivity of the changes more frequently than others.

Paranoid Profile

The behavior of paranoid patients during LSD-assisted therapy reflects their unresolved tendency towards delusional negative interpretations of reality more intensely. Grof comments that his observations of patients with a paranoid personality profile can likely confirm a connection between homosexuality and paranoid behavior. Latent homosexual feelings may surface and be projected onto the therapist of the same gender. In male patients, this realization of latent homosexuality can be accompanied by strong fears and panic attacks. Particularly, this can be aggravated by experiencing sexual feelings toward the opposite gender. Grof reports frequently observing feedback from male patients stating that during LSD-25 therapy, they felt a female body and experienced clitoral and vaginal orgasms. He also notes similar occurrences in female patients, where they described experiencing male-type orgasms. However, such cases were much less frequent in male patients.

Psychopathic Profile

Stanislav Grof has written extensively about how LSD therapy can significantly alter the psychopathic symptoms of patients. However, the experiences these individuals undergo during LSD-25 sessions are often intense and distressing. Patients frequently recount experiences of being in hell and enduring various tortures. The intensity of these experiences may prompt the patient to request that the session be interrupted (for which the drug naloxone is typically used). Unbearable mental anguish can transition into shifts to alternative personalities. For instance, Grof describes a case in which he worked with LSD-25 with a woman who had an antisocial personality, had been incarcerated multiple times, engaged in heavy drug use, and identified as a lesbian. Her symptoms of antisocial behavior closely resembled the concept of a psychopathic personality profile. During the therapy, the patient shifted into an alternative personality, identifying herself as a devil and threatening Grof, promising him many troubles if he didn't stop helping her. This part of her personality dissipated after the LSD session ended. Subsequently, Grof observed significant changes in her. She stopped using drugs, managed to find adequate social work, and even established heterosexual relationships. However, unfortunately, she couldn't maintain them for long and returned to homosexual relationships. Grof admitted that after this incident, he started considering having a Christian crucifix present during sessions with patients, just in case. Similar processes, in different forms, can occur in other psychopathic patients.

True psychopathic individuals are incapable of experiencing guilt and shame. However, when we talk about a psychopathic accent, the feeling of guilt and shame may not arise in certain life situations.

For example, in relationships with the opposite sex, in business relationships, etc. On a physiological level, psychopathy is manifested by weak activity in the anterior and posterior cingulate gyrus, which is directly related to the capacity for empathy and compassion. It seems that LSD-25 is capable of awakening these brain regions. During an LSD session, the psychopath, in a way, comes face to face with their conscience, which they have suppressed for a long time or their entire life. The various "hellish" experiences they go through likely reflect their actions. Thus, the integration of personality fragments takes place.

According to the current legislation in most countries worldwide, psychotherapists are not allowed to conduct LSD sessions with their patients. However, thanks to Stanislav Grof's developed technique of holotropic breathing, which is completely legal and recognized in many countries, we can observe effects similar to those of LSD sessions. A similar pattern emerges when psychopathic patients, undergoing deep breathing processes, often confront a very difficult and unpleasant integration, which unequivocally indicates the fragmented nature of their personality. Unlike schizophrenic personality disorder, where fragmented parts can simultaneously exist within consciousness, the psychopath is only aware of one aggressive part. The sacrificial part is constantly projected onto other people to make them feel good, continuously causing pain and suffering to others.

Obsessive-Compulsive Profile

Grof describes working with LSD-25 and obsessive-compulsive patients as quite challenging. These patients exhibit a high level of resistance to the substance. It seems that they can withstand doses of over 500 mcg, only reporting some unpleasant sensations in their bodies. Sometimes, multiple LSD sessions are required for the patient to weaken their psychological defenses and allow unconscious material to be released calmly.

Grof also reports that increasing the dosage usually leads to no significant results. He observed a case where a patient was given a dose of 15,000 mcg intramuscularly, which had little effect. As we can see, increasing the dosage is ineffective. Psychiatrists have found a dosage limit of 400–500 mcg. If a patient does not respond to this dose, further increases are unlikely to have any effect. Obsessive-compulsive patients express numerous anxieties and fears about the upcoming session, which, of course, creates strong tension during the LSD session and hinders the free expression of unconscious material. The patient may literally struggle against the effects of the substance. There is a strong need for total self-control. Visual sensations are almost absent, and bodily representations are more common. Various complaints such as headaches, nausea, sweating, and unpleasant sensations are frequent. The session becomes a constant inner struggle, leading to profound fatigue.

This self-struggle has a pronounced psychodynamic aspect, which can shed light on the underlying cause of the symptom, rooted in powerful resistance and rejection of one of the parental figures. Often, it is the father figure.

Schizoid Profile

Resistance from schizoid individuals towards psychedelic work can be very strong. The level of resistance may resemble that of patients with obsessive-compulsive symptoms.

Epileptoid Profile

Individuals with an epileptoid character are capable of strongly unveiling unconscious processes, which is reminiscent of the demonstrative profile but without excessive exaggeration of effects. They often experience greater comfort working with higher doses. If we specifically discuss epilepsy as a disease, working with epileptic patients can be problematic because LSD-25 can trigger an uncontrollable series of epileptoid seizures that are difficult to control. This is why working with such patients can be life-threatening.

Schizophrenic Profile

LSD-25 has been tested on patients suffering from schizophrenia by various psychiatrists in different countries. In Europe, there were even specialized clinics dedicated to treating schizophrenic patients with this drug and similar ones in terms of quality. Numerous studies have been conducted, showing that the drug could create positive dynamics for some patients.

Manic-Depressive Profile

Symptoms of manic-depressive psychosis, like symptoms of depression, are closely related to serotonin secretion in the human brain. In such disorders, serotonin secretion significantly decreases. LSD-25 has the ability to activate serotonin receptors in the human brain. Therefore, the use of LSD in such patients can cause significant remissions. Formally, depression is the symptom that was well addressed during the clinical trials of LSD-25. LSD sessions are often accompanied by strong euphoria, laughter, and joy in depressive patients. Some observations have led to the assumption that even a single administration can induce complete remission.

It has also been found that LSD affects patients with exogenous and endogenous depression differently. Grof describes how patients with exogenous depression interact deeply on a profound level. They delve deeply into a wide range of biographical material that holds psychodynamic significance in relation to the symptom. On the other hand, patients suffering from endogenous depression often fixate on specific, profound primal emotions that form the basis of their depression. These patients are at risk of experiencing a temporary exacerbation of symptoms after an LSD session. Grof comments that his observations align with the experiments of Danish psychiatrist Arendsen-Hinsh, who was one of the pioneers in the clinical application of LSD-25.

Afterword

It is important to draw the reader's attention to the fact that currently, various forms of psychedelic therapy are not legal in most countries worldwide. Therefore, the information we present here is based on the accumulated data from our colleagues in the United States and European countries before the prohibition on the use of the described methods of psychotherapeutic work. It is also essential to emphasize that the information in this chapter regarding the use and application of psychedelic substances is strictly commented on in a clinical medical context and has no relevance to their non-professional use outside of medical institutions.

A Brief Message from the Author

Mastering complex psychotherapeutic theories and practices can be a challenging journey. By sharing your experience with this book, you can guide others who are on the same path. Your review could inspire someone to take the next step in deepening their knowledge and applying these insights to make meaningful changes in their life.

Thank you for your support and for taking the time to share your thoughts! Your feedback helps us refine our offerings and empowers others in their pursuit of mastering psychotherapy. If this book has been valuable to you, I'd be grateful if you could take a moment to leave a review. **Your positive rating would mean a lot!**

To share your feedback, simply scan the QR code or click the link below:

psychemaster.com/recommends/review-psychedelic-therapy

Bibliography

1. Grof, S. (1980). LSD Psychotherapy. (Translated by Georgiy Valeriyevich). [Self-published, available in electronic libraries]

2. Grof, S. (2009). LSD: Doorway to the Numinous: Groundbreaking Psychedelic Research into the Realms of the Human Unconscious.

3. Hagenbach, D., & Werthmüller, L. (2013). Mystic Chemist: The Life of Albert Hofmann and His Discovery of LSD. Synergetic Press. ISBN 978-090779146-1.

4. Hofmann, A. (1979). "LSD, My Problem Child."

5. Roberts, A. (2008). Albion Dreaming: A Popular History of LSD in Britain. Marshall Cavendish, U.K. ISBN 978-190573 6270/1905736274.

6. Shulgin, A., & Shulgin, A. (1991). "PiHKAL: A Chemical Love Story." Berkeley: Transform Press. ISBN 0-9630096-0-5.

7. Shulgin, A., & Shulgin, A. (1997). "TiHKAL: The Continuation." Berkeley: Transform Press. ISBN 0-9630096-9-9.

8. Winkelman, M. (2007). "Shamanic Guidelines for Psychedelic Medicine." In Winkelman, M., & Roberts, T. B. (Eds.), Psychedelic Medicine: New Evidence for Hallucinogenic Substances as Treatments. Westport, CT: Praeger Publishers. ISBN 978-0-275-99023-7.

9. Grof, S. (1994). Realms of the Human Unconscious: Observations from LSD Research. Moscow: MTM. (240 pages)

10. Grof, S. (2000). Beyond the Brain: Birth, Death, and Transcendence in Psychotherapy (3rd ed.). Moscow: Institute of Transpersonal Psychology, Institute of Psychotherapy Publishing. (504 pages) ISBN 5-93509-004-X, 5-89939-012-3. Available in libraries.

11. Grof, S. (2013). Holotropic Breathwork: A New Approach to Self-Exploration and Therapy. Moscow: Ganga. (352 pages) (Transpersonal Psychology) ISBN 978-5-906154-38-5.

12. Leuner, H. (1996). Catathymic Imagery. Translated by Ya. L. Obukhova. Moscow: "Eidos."

13. Leuner, H. (1996). Fundamentals of Depth Psychological Symbolism. Translated by Ya. L. Obukhova. Journal of Practical Psychologist, No. 3, 4.

14. Leuner, H. (1996). Directed Affective Imagery. In: Anthology of Depth Psychology, compiled by L. A. Hegai. Moscow: CheRo. Vol. 1, pp. 154-176. (C. G. Jung and Modern Psychoanalysis) (5000 copies) ISBN 5-88711-008-2.

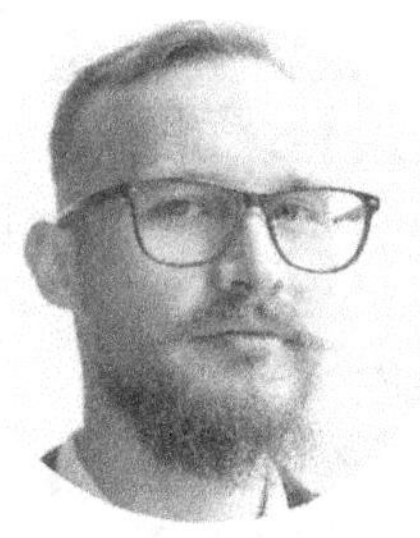

About the Author

Dr. **Artem Kudelia**, a psychologist with a PhD and a practicing therapist, has extensive expertise in integrative approaches. He possesses comprehensive knowledge of a wide range of psychotherapeutic methods, including humanistic and existential theories, as well as the practical application of cognitive-behavioral therapy (CBT) to effectively address issues such as anxiety, depression, obsessive thoughts, compulsions, social phobias, and complex emotions. His books are valuable resources for professionals and individuals interested in managing their mental health. In addition to managing symptoms, he helps his clients toward self-actualization in various aspects of their lives, including social, career, and personal aspects.

You can connect with me on:

- 🔗 https://facebook.com/psyche.masters
- 🔗 https://instagram.com/psyche.masters
- 🔗 https://threads.net/@psyche.masters
- 🔗 https://youtube.com/@psyche.masters
- 🔗 https://tiktok.com/@psyche.masters
- 🔗 https://pinterest.com/psychemasters

Subscribe to my newsletter:

- ✉ https://psychemaster.com/early-reader-signup

Also by Artem Kudelia PhD

The ***Psychology & Psychotherapy Theories & Practices*** series offers a detailed examination of the history, theoretical foundations, and practical applications of fundamental approaches in psychotherapy. It is an indispensable resource for psychologists, medical professionals, psychology students, and anyone interested in understanding these complex subjects.

Additionally, the ***Cognitive Behavioral Therapy Self-Help Guide: 15 Steps to Mental Health*** series provides actionable guidance for overcoming various psychological challenges, such as anxiety, depression, excessive anger, obsessive thoughts, compulsions, social phobias, health anxiety, and intricate emotional struggles. These topics were chosen because many individuals facing these challenges often lack awareness of the underlying dynamics. By gaining insight into these processes, individuals can make informed decisions about seeking help, reinforcing the idea that knowledge is a powerful tool for personal empowerment.

Together, these series offer invaluable resources for those interested in psychology, whether for academic study or personal development, by providing comprehensive insights and practical tools that contribute to improved mental well-being.

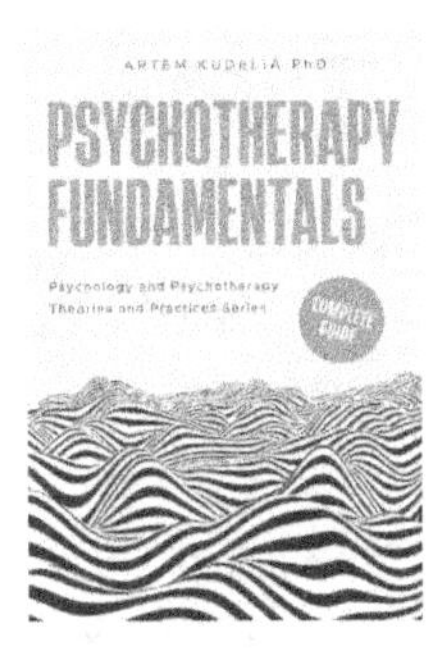

**Psychotherapy Fundamentals
Complete Guide**

Are you struggling to understand complex psychotherapeutic theories?

Psychotherapy Fundamentals: Complete Guide simplifies the intricate world of psychotherapy, making it accessible and actionable for those interested in self-discovery, self-education, and readers with a wide range of interests.

❤ **Imagine confidently navigating psychotherapeutic real-world scenarios with ease.**

This book is your *comprehensive roadmap to achieving a deep and practical understanding of psychotherapy.* You'll learn to simplify complex theories and integrate them effectively into your life and practice.

Gain a comprehensive understanding of various therapeutic approaches, including *provocative* therapy, *humanistic* therapy, *somatic* therapy, *existential* therapy, *drama* therapy, *psychedelic* and *post-psychedelic* therapy, *anti-psychiatric* therapy, and *integrative* therapy. Each chapter delves into the key themes and methods of these psychotherapy modalities, broadening the horizons for those interested in self-discovery, self-education, and lifelong learning.

https://books2read.com/Psychotherapy-Fundamentals

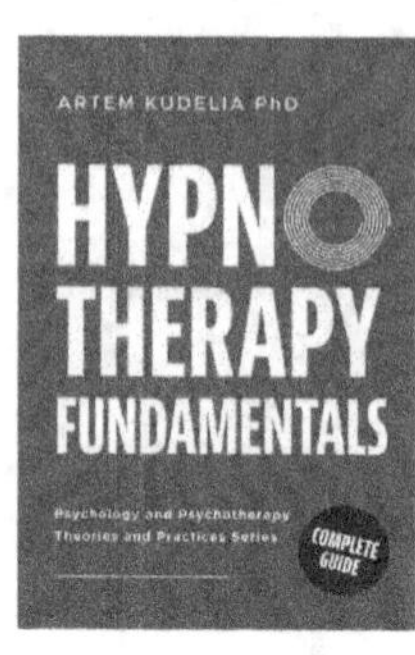

**Hypnotherapy Fundamentals
Complete Guide**

Are you ready to uncover the secrets of hypnotherapy?

This comprehensive guide immerses you in the **theory** *and history of hypnosis*, providing a solid foundation for understanding the principles underlying hypnotherapy.

Explore the various techniques and approaches used in *hypnotherapy* **training** through **practice exercises**, including the art of *suggestion* and deepening *hypnotic trance states*, the creation of therapeutic propositions, and the utilization of the power of the subconscious mind.

Learn how to effectively apply *hypnotherapy techniques* to address a wide range of issues, from managing stress and anxiety to overcoming phobias and habits.

Gain an understanding of the transformative potential of hypnosis and its applications for personal growth and well-being.

Unlock the secrets of harnessing the power of the mind and creating positive changes in yourself and others.

https://books2read.com/Hypnotherapy-Fundamentals

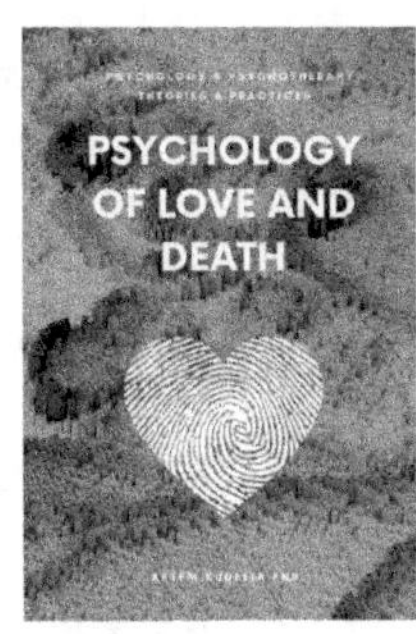

**Psychology of Love & Death
Therapeutic Path to Fundamental Balance
in Life and Relationships**

*How to Achieve Fundamental Balance in Life
and Relationships?*

Explore dualistic nature of human consciousness, along with the profound impact of seeking balance between fundamental continuums of *love and death*, *instinct and spirituality*, *masculinity and femininity* in shaping our experiences and relationships.

Explore the psychopathological profiles and manifestations of love and death, including profiles such as hysteria, paranoia, psychopathy, and others.

Uncover different types of love, from eros to agape, and study the *three-component Theory of Love*.

Familiarize yourself with *real-life psychotherapy cases* that illustrate the complexities of love, death, and therapy and gain *valuable insights* into the human experience and its challenges.

https://books2read.com/Psychology-of-Love-and-Death

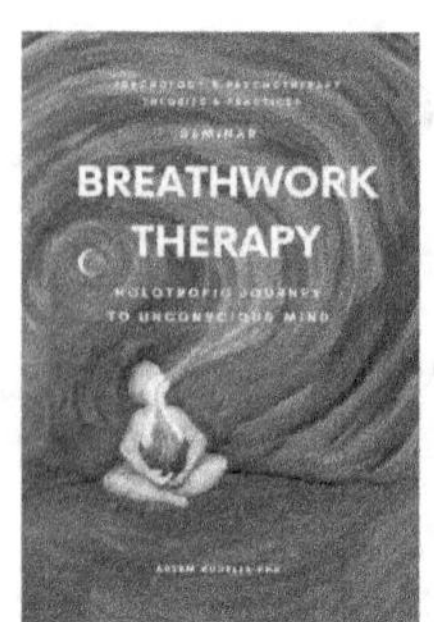

**Breathwork Therapy Seminar
Holotropic Journey to Unconscious Mind
Secrets**

Tap Into the Wisdom of Transpersonal Psychology!

This book is the transcript of a seminar that addresses the profound questions of *subconsciousness*, offering a unique perspective on personal growth and healing.

Gain profound insights into the workings of your mind and explore the mysteries of human consciousness.

Access practical exercises and *techniques* to facilitate personal growth, healing, and self-awareness through *breathwork*.

Written for seekers of self-awareness, psychology enthusiasts, and anyone curious about the depths of the human mind.

Explore the integration of spirituality and psychology, uncovering your inner potential.

▽

https://books2read.com/Breathwork-Therapy

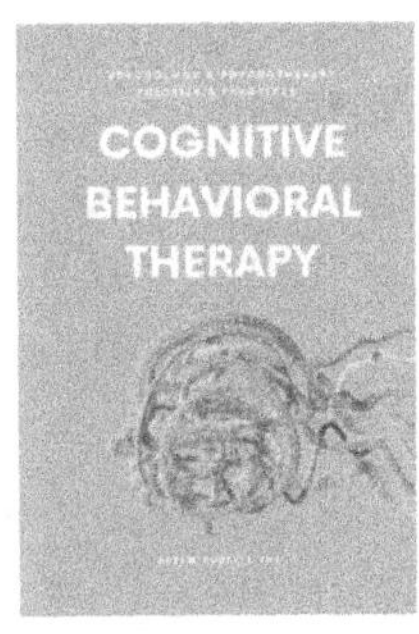

**Cognitive Behavioral Therapy
Managing Anxiety and Depression**

Explore the roots of anxiety and learn why it's a fundamental aspect of the human experience.

An in-depth exploration of *Panic Disorder*, addressing the irrational fears associated with it.

Examine the nuances of *Social Anxiety* and its impact on personal and professional spheres.

Dive into the world of *Obsessive-Compulsive Disorder*, unraveling its complexities.

Understand the genetic predispositions and learn effective strategies to manage obsessions and compulsions.

Explore *PTSD* from its roots to its biological manifestations. Delve into the trauma cycles, and discover therapeutic techniques for stabilization and overcoming trauma.

Grasp the degrees of *Depression*, from mild to severe, debunking common myths.

https://books2read.com/Cognitive-Behavioral-Therapy

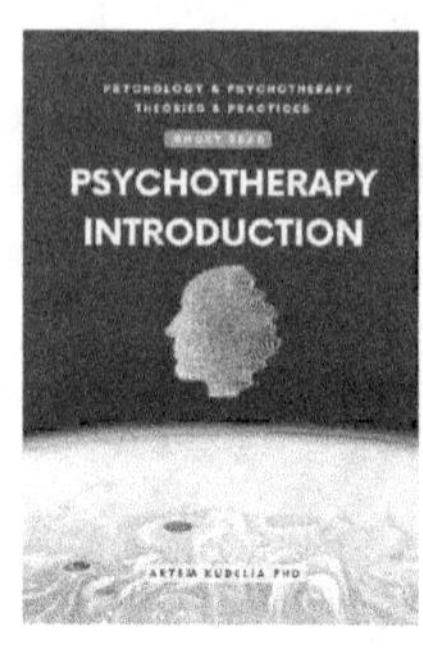

**Psychotherapy
Introduction to Healing Vectors**

Do you want to understand the variety of methods of psychotherapy and choose the one that is best for you?

In the vast world of psycho-technologies, there are numerous methods of psychotherapy that encompass a wide range of *personality theories* and concepts.

Drawing upon an integral framework, the book maps out the complex *landscape of psychotherapy*, encompassing vectors such as *psychoanalytic, hypnotic, provocative, humanistic, behavioral, existential, transpersonal, cognitive, somatic, psychodramatic* and *psychedelic* therapies, among many others.

This book will provide you with valuable knowledge that will allow you to choose the most suitable therapeutic path for specific circumstances and personality types.

https://books2read.com/Psychotherapy-Introduction

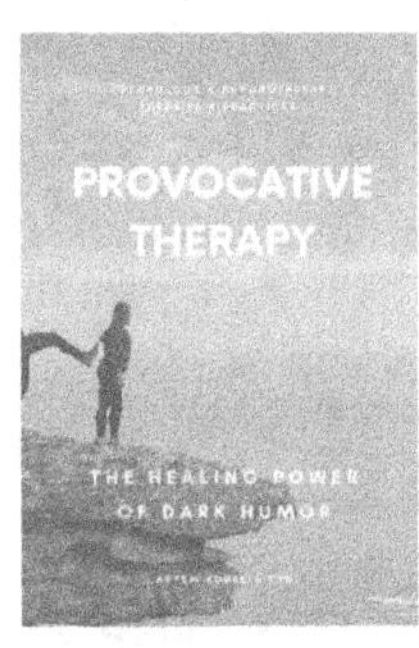

Provocative Therapy
The Healing Power of Dark Humor

Who said that psychotherapy can't be hilariously funny?

Explore innovative ideas about the power of humor in psychotherapy and coaching.

Uncover the archetypal foundation of Provocative Therapy inspired by the myths of the Trickster and the Holy Fool.

Delve into the transformational potential of *Group Provocative Psychotherapy* and the important rules that define successful group dynamics.

Explore the effectiveness of *Provocative Coaching* and its focus points.

Dive into the fascinating world of *Provocative Drama* and its role in therapeutic interventions.

Explore the *pathopsychological profiles*, including *hysteroid, paranoid, psychopathic, obsessive-compulsive, schizoid, epileptoid, schizophrenic,* and *manic-depressive* profiles.

https://books2read.com/Provocative-Therapy

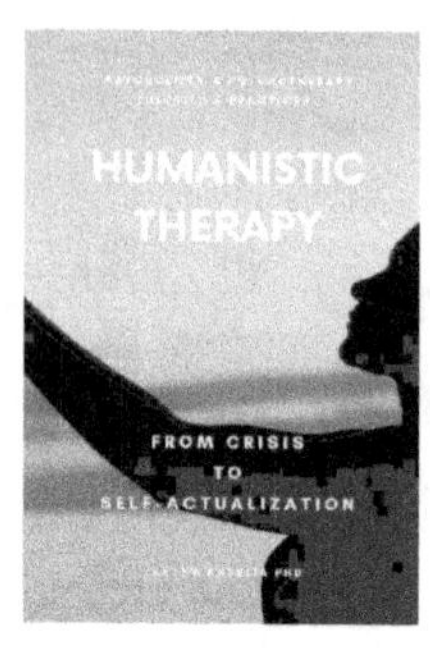

Humanistic Therapy
From Crisis to Self-Actualization

Do you want to explore a world where people are seen as unique holistic systems with infinite potential waiting to be discovered?

Immerse yourself in the theories and practices of humanistic therapy and explore the *transformative path from crisis to self-actualization.*

Unlike psychoanalysis, which focuses on internal complexes and personal traumas, humanistic therapy emphasizes the *study and development of positive personality qualities.*

Humanistic philosophy has also influenced fields such as *education*, promoting *empathy* and *support* as the foundation of learning.

This holistic approach recognizes the *interconnectedness of mind, body, and spirit* and seeks to stimulate personal *growth* and *well-being.*

Take the first step towards self-awareness, personal growth, and a more fulfilling existence.

https://books2read.com/Humanistic-Therapy

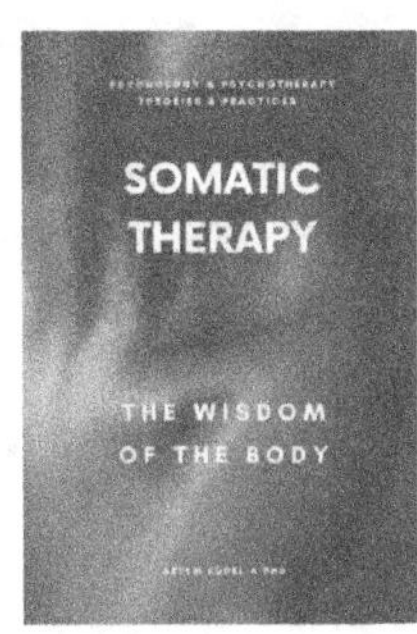

**Somatic Therapy
The Wisdom of the Body**

Would you like to establish a connection with your body and access the source of wisdom?

Unleash the transformative power of *somatic therapy* and embark on a journey of *self-discovery* and *healing*.

Explore the profound connection between the *mind and body.*

Discover the *seven levels of muscular armor* and their connection to specific emotions such as sadness, anger, and fear.

By exploring different body segments, you will unlock *powerful techniques* for releasing pent-up emotions and promoting harmony throughout the organism. From *eye movements* and *jaw exercises* to *deep breathing* and *body movements*, this book offers *practical methods* for *accessing the wisdom of the body* and *restoring emotional balance.*

Acquire unique knowledge about *healing after birth trauma and psychosomatic medicine.*

https://books2read.com/Somatic-Therapy

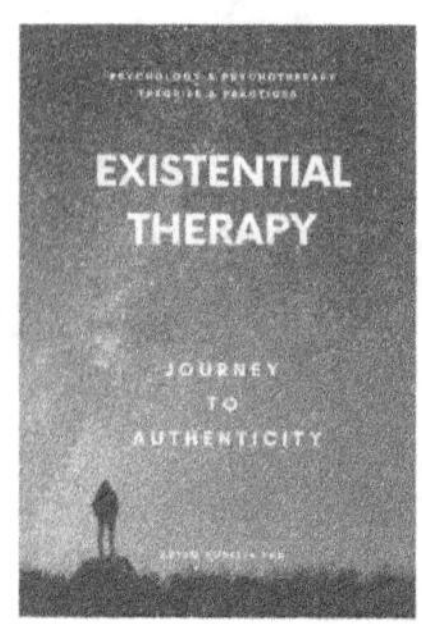

**Existential Therapy
Journey to Authenticity**

*Do you want to know who you really are?
What is your personal meaning of existence?*

Embark on a *transformative journey* to uncover your *true essence* and embrace the *principles* of existential therapy.

Explore the rich philosophical roots of *existential psychotherapy* and find your path to *personal authenticity*.

Explore key themes such as *freedom, responsibility, meaning,* and *choice*, and learn to courageously and authentically navigate the complexities of existence.

This book provides *practical ideas and techniques* for *applying the principles of existential therapy* to your own life.

Gain a deep *understanding* of your *values, beliefs,* and *desires,* and learn to *embrace uncertainty* and *transform* life's *challenges* into *opportunities* for *growth* and *self-discovery.*

https://books2read.com/Existential-Therapy

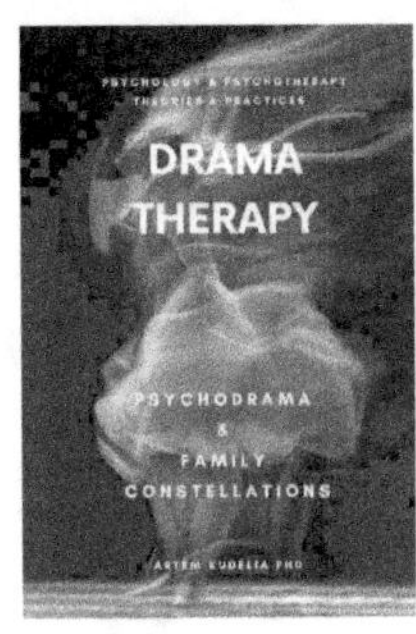

**Drama Therapy
Potential of Psychodrama and Family Constellations**

Explore the unique world of drama therapeutic approach!

Therapeutic model of intervention that encompasses 12 *powerful speech patterns* capable of significantly *influencing conscious and unconscious processes.*

Through *psychodramatic techniques* and *family constellations,* you will *gain practical knowledge* to enhance your therapeutic practice.

Addressing a wide spectrum of *psychopathological profiles,* including *hysteria, paranoia,* and *obsessive-compulsive disorders,* this book equips you with effective dramatherapeutic activities and psychodynamic exercises.

It serves as a *comprehensive guide* to *crisis intervention, counseling theory,* and *strategies for addiction rehabilitation.*

Gain an understanding of the right hemisphere and the *neuroscience* underlying drama therapy, and learn to *navigate complex emotional situations* with *understanding* and *acceptance.*

https://books2read.com/Drama-Therapy-Constellations

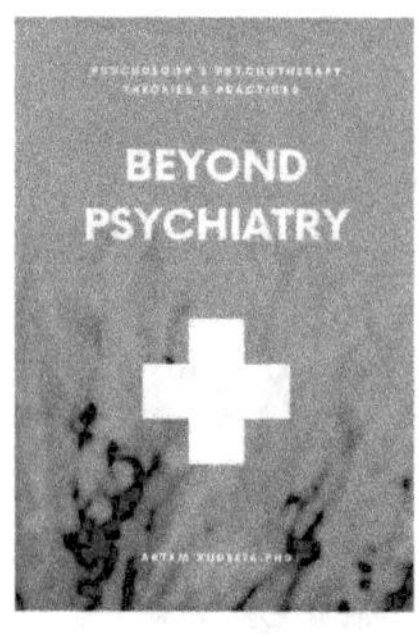

Beyond Psychiatry
Exploring Anti-Psychiatry Method

Challenge traditional psychiatry and psychotherapy!

This book presents an *alternative to conventional* ideas of normalcy and offers a *fresh perspective on psychological disorders*, inviting readers to question existing paradigms.

Delve deeper into *psychopathological profiles* and *anti-psychiatric* forms of psychotherapy, examining various profiles including *hysteria, paranoia, psychopathy*, and more.

Gain an understanding of the intersection of psychotherapy and existential philosophy, *challenging the myth of mental illness* within families.

Explore the *treatment of psychosis, trauma,* and *emotional disorders from a holistic perspective.*

https://books2read.com/Beyond-Psychiatry

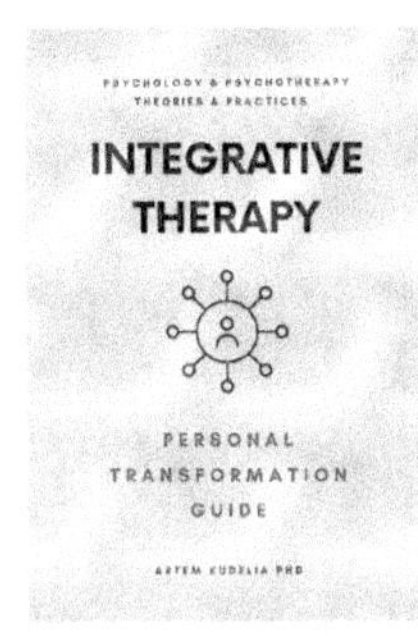

**Integrative Therapy
Personal Transformation Guide**

Discover the Power of Integrative Therapy and Embark on a Journey of Personal Transformation!

This book challenges traditional divisions in *therapeutic approaches* and explores the potential of *combining multiple vectors* to create a *comprehensive and integrated therapeutic system.*

Immerse yourself in the world of *neuro-linguistic programming* (NLP), *cognitive styles, neurological levels,* and *integral philosophy,* among other concepts.

Explore practical methodologies such as *shifting negative thinking, creating rapport,* and using linguistic patterns to facilitate positive change.

Unlock the transformative *power of anchors, changing personal history* and *submodalities.*

Gain an understanding of maps of the world and the *metamodel* for *effective communication.*

https://books2read.com/Integrative-Therapy

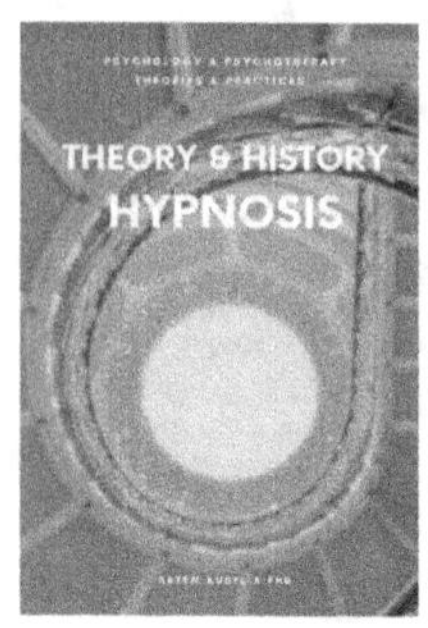

Theory & History of Hypnosis
Exploring Altered State of Mind in Trance

Immerse yourself in the fascinating world of hypnosis and explore the history and theory of altered states of consciousness!

This book sheds light on *historical trance practices* and the *role of shamanism*, tracing its influence on *modern psychospiritual orientations*.

Discover the benefits of this book by exploring the *history of trance practices and hypnotherapy.*

Explore the *evolution* of *shamanism*, its connection to *religion*, and its pre-religious *philosophy*, which offered deep insights into the structure of the universe and the mysteries of the spiritual world.

Discover various *hypnotic phenomena* and *states of consciousness* that can be induced in a trance state.

Explore their potential applications in *psychotherapeutic practice*, from *pain management* to the *treatment of depression.*

Learn techniques such as *self-hypnosis, deep trance induction*, and *guided healing visualizations.*

https://books2read.com/Theory-and-History-of-Hypnosis

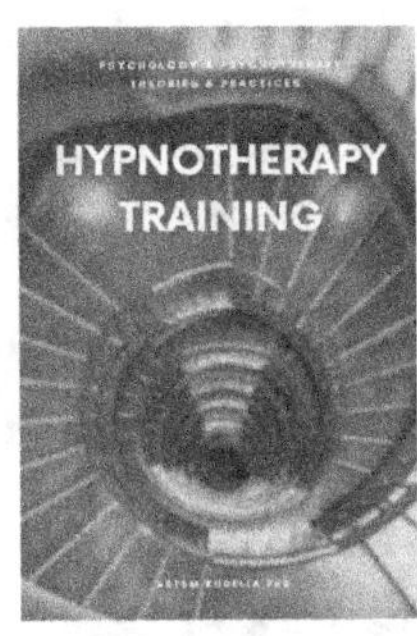

**Hypnotherapy Training
A Guide for Practicing Hypnotherapists**

Uncover the secrets of hypnotherapy and improve your practical hypnosis skills!

This book explores *techniques* and *practical skills* for hypnotherapists.

Dive into the depths of the *subconscious* and discover the *transformative potential* of hypnotherapy.

Discover the benefits of this book, which delves into key topics and approaches in *hypnotherapy training.*

Explore developed techniques, including rapport-building practices and the use of matching postures, movements, and breathing with the client.

Engage in exercises that enable the attainment of different trance levels and explore the motives of trance and their application in psychotherapy.

Gain an understanding of different styles and orientations of hypnotic work, from hypnoanalytic and suggestive to behavioral and transpersonal.

https://books2read.com/Hypnotherapy-Training

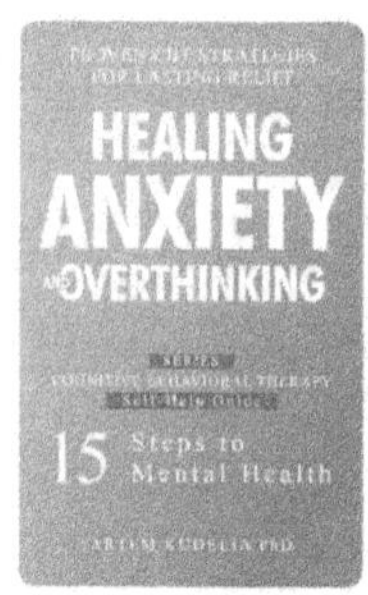

Healing Anxiety and Overthinking
Proven CBT Strategies for Lasting Relief

Are you exhausted from the relentless cycle of anxiety and overthinking?

Discover the 15-step program that will transform your mental health and bring peace of mind.

Millions of adults struggle with anxiety and overthinking, feeling trapped in a cycle of worry and stress. But it doesn't have to be this way. *"Healing Anxiety and Overthinking: Proven CBT Strategies for Lasting Relief"* offers a comprehensive guide to breaking free from the grip of anxiety using practical, proven **Cognitive Behavioral Therapy (CBT)** strategies.

❤️ *Imagine waking up every day with a clear mind, free from the constant barrage of anxious thoughts*

This book is your roadmap to achieving that transformation in just 15 steps. You'll learn to understand the nature of your anxiety, identify its triggers, and apply effective techniques to manage and overcome it.

Take Control of Your Mental Health

Don't let anxiety and overthinking rule your life. With *"Healing Anxiety and Overthinking,"* you'll gain the tools and confidence to achieve peace of mind and live the life you deserve.

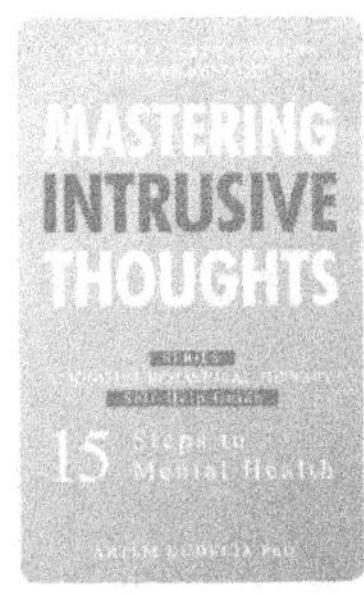

**Mastering Intrusive Thoughts
Practical CBT Techniques for Managing OCD**

*Is **OCD** ruling your life with intrusive thoughts and compulsions?*

Take back control with scientifically-proven CBT techniques designed to help you regain peace of mind.

Millions of adults struggle with obsessive-compulsive disorder (OCD), caught in a relentless cycle of intrusive thoughts and compulsive behaviors. "Mastering Intrusive Thoughts" is your step-by-step guide to breaking free from the grip of OCD using practical, evidence-based Cognitive Behavioral Therapy (CBT) techniques.

❤ *Picture yourself waking up with a calm, focused mind, no longer burdened by the constant anxiety of unwanted thoughts.*

In this book, Dr. Artem Kudelia offers a clear and actionable path to mastering your thoughts in 15 manageable steps. Whether you're new to CBT or have tried other methods without success, this guide provides the tools you need to finally achieve relief.

✔ **Take the First Step Towards Mental Freedom**

You'll gain the knowledge and confidence to conquer your **OCD** and reclaim your peace of mind.

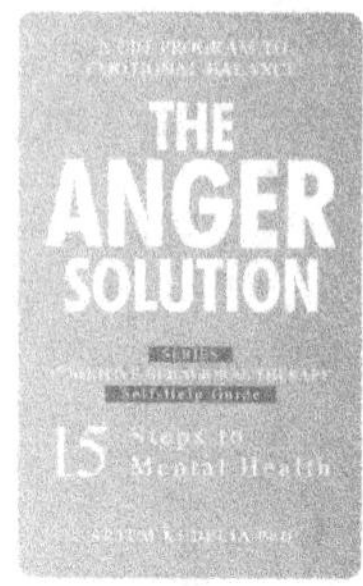

The Anger Solution
A CBT Program for Emotional Balance

Are you tired of living with persistent anger and overwhelming stress?

Discover a practical, 15-step program designed to bring lasting peace and transform your emotional health.

Millions of adults struggle with anger and stress, feeling trapped in a cycle of frustration and tension. But it doesn't have to be this way. "The Anger Solution" offers a comprehensive guide to breaking free from the grip of anger using practical, proven Cognitive Behavioral Therapy (CBT) strategies.

❤️ *Imagine waking up every day with a calm mind, free from the constant barrage of anger and stress.*

This book is your roadmap to achieving that transformation. With clear, actionable steps, you'll learn to understand the nature of your anger, identify its triggers, and apply effective techniques to manage and overcome it.

✔ **Take Control of Your Emotional Health**

With "The Anger Solution," you'll gain the tools and confidence to achieve emotional balance and live the life you deserve.

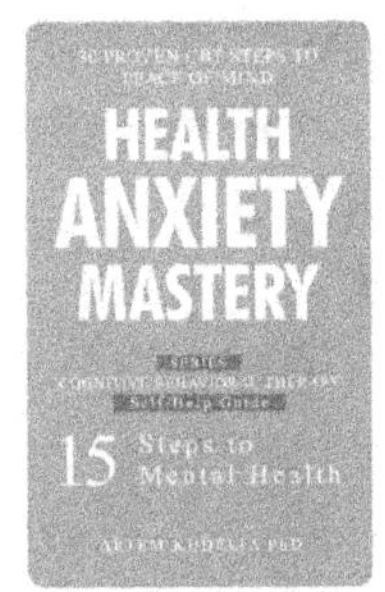

Health Anxiety Mastery
30 Proven CBT Steps to Peace of Mind

Is health anxiety controlling your life with constant worry and fear?

Regain peace of mind with proven CBT techniques designed to help you overcome health-related anxiety and reclaim control.

Millions of people struggle with health anxiety, trapped in a cycle of physical symptoms, endless reassurance-seeking, and intrusive thoughts about their well-being. *"Health Anxiety Mastery"* offers a clear, step-by-step approach to breaking free from these patterns using practical, evidence-based Cognitive Behavioral Therapy (CBT) techniques.

❤ **Imagine waking up each day calm and confident, no longer overwhelmed by fear and obsessive thoughts about your health.**

In this book, you'll find 30 actionable steps to help you reduce anxiety, challenge limiting beliefs, and develop healthier thought patterns. Whether you're just beginning your journey or have tried other approaches without success, these practical tools will guide you toward lasting relief.

✔ **Start Your Journey to Balanced Mental Health**

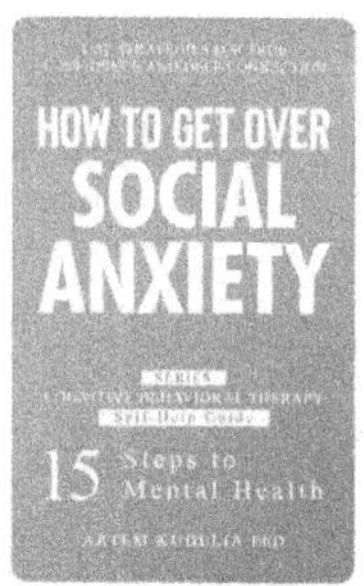

**How to Get Over Social Anxiety
CBT Strategies for True Confidence and
Deep Connection**

*What if 15 proven steps could free you from
social anxiety and help you connect?*

Uncover a 15-step CBT program to overcome fear, stop avoidance, and build true self-confidence. Millions struggle with social anxiety, but you don't have to face it alone. This guide provides a clear, evidence-based path to transforming your social life and connecting authentically.

♥ **Imagine engaging in conversations fearlessly and forming genuine relationships free from judgment or rejection.**

With insights from proven cognitive-behavioral techniques and relatable examples, this book offers the practical tools and encouragement needed to face your fears and succeed socially.

✔ **Begin Your Journey to Confidence**

Start transforming fear into connection and reclaim control of your social life with *"How to Get Over Social Anxiety."*

Discover More by Artem Kudelia
Scan the QR code or click the link to access his author page and full collection. Each book provides detailed insights and practical guidance, exemplifying his contributions to psychology and psychotherapy.

books2read.com/Artem-Kudelia-PhD